LIVING WITH ASTHMA

DR ROBERT YOUNGSON MB, ChB, DTM&H, DO, FRC Ophth, a former medical consultant, is now a full-time writer. He is the author of twenty popular medical and science books, including *Coping with Hay Fever* and *Coping with Eczema* (both Sheldon Press, 1995) and has also written extensively on medical topics for *Reader's Digest* and *Good Housekeeping* books. He has made many radio broadcasts and has appeared on television.

Overcoming Common Problems

LIVING WITH ASTHMA

Dr Robert Youngson

sheldon PRESS

First published in Great Britain in 1995 by
Sheldon Press, SPCK, Marylebone Road, London NW1 4DU

Second impression 1998

British Library Cataloguing-in-Publication Data
A catalogue record for this book is available from the British Library

ISBN 0–85969–724–4

Photoset by Deltatype Ltd, Ellesmere Port, Cheshire
Printed in Great Britain by Biddles Ltd, Guildford and King's Lynn

Contents

For Muriel

Introduction

Asthma is one of the commonest of the conditions affecting people of all ages. In Britain, nearly three million people – some 5 per cent of the population – have asthma, and, as a result of worsening atmospheric pollution and other factors, it is getting steadily commoner. More people are becoming asthmatic and people with asthma are having more attacks. The number of asthma attacks has doubled since 1974. Children are affected about twice as often as adults. About one child in seven now suffers from asthma. Much the same applies to the rest of Europe. In the United States and Australia, it is estimated that about 5 per cent of adults and 10 per cent of children suffer from asthma.

Asthma varies greatly in severity and, because most attacks are comparatively mild, it is often thought to be a minor disorder. This is not so. Asthma is a treacherous condition that can go quickly out of control. You should never underestimate its dangers. In Britain alone, over 2,000 people die from asthma every year, and many of these are people who have not considered themselves to be severely affected. All the experts are concerned at the lack of knowledge of the subject among asthmatics and their parents. Failure to understand the principles of treatment and to recognize the danger signs commonly leads to undertreatment and dangerous delay in seeking medical help when this is urgently needed.

There is nothing like real life for bringing home important points. So this book contains a number of case histories illustrating these essential features of the story. It would not do to publish details from real clinical notes, so these cases are presented in fictional form. All the events described in these cases, however, actually happened.

If you or your child are asthmatic, you owe it to yourself to know as much as possible about asthma. You will find everything you need to know in this book.

1

What is asthma?

The earliest known written reference to asthma appears in 1398 in an encyclopedia called *De Proprietatibus Rerum* (On the Properties of Things) written in Latin by the English scholar Bartholomaeus Anglicus. In his 19-volume work, Bartholomaeus tried to cover all the knowledge of his time, including science and medicine. This book was translated into English by John of Trevisa and was printed in 1495. It was one of the first best-sellers and was greatly influential in Tudor England. Referring to asthma, Trevisa's translation says, 'Dyffy-culte and hardnes of brethynge hight Asma'. Bartholomaeus recognized that there were different conditions that produced asthma-like symptoms, and suggested that there were 'Thre manere of Asmyes'. The word comes from the Greek *asthma*, meaning 'to breathe hard'.

In 1578 the English botanist and antiquary Henry Lyte published a translation of the French *Cruydboeck* of Rembert Dodoens, under the title *A niewe Herball or Historie of Plantes*, in which he referred to a remedy for 'The shortnesse of breath called asthma'. After that there were increasing references which gradually refined the meaning of the word until, by the middle of the nineteenth century, the term was generally used in its more restricted modern sense. All this indicates that, throughout the ages, countless millions of people must have suffered from disorders that make breathing difficult. No doubt some of these were conditions due to other chest disorders, but a great many of them must have been the same distressing condition suffered by so many asthmatic people today.

Before answering the question posed by the heading of this chapter, it is necessary to explain a few basic facts. You will not be able to understand asthma fully until you know about these. Everyone concerned directly or indirectly concerned with asthma should be aware of them.

The importance of oxygen

Oxygen – the important gas that makes up about 20 per cent of the atmosphere – is a vital necessity. We can live for weeks without food and for days without water, but if we are totally deprived of oxygen for even a few minutes we will die. Because of this, nature has arranged that whenever we get short of oxygen, we forget everything else and concentrate wholly on getting air. Not only are we very much aware of the necessity to breathe, but we also experience some strong and very unpleasant warning signals which are the body's way of telling us that the top priority is to get oxygen. Only those who have experienced a severe asthmatic attack can be fully aware of the distress involved in this and of how easy it is to yield to panic. Only these people can have a full, emotional appreciation of what it is like to breathe easily and freely and without any special effort – something the rest of us take for granted.

How we get our oxygen

If our bodies are to be able to use oxygen it must get into our bloodstreams. Here is how it does so. By moving our ribs upwards and outwards, and the muscular floor of the chest (the *diaphragm*) downwards, we draw air into our lungs through nose or mouth – preferably the former. This air then passes through the voice box (*larynx*) and the air tubes. The main air tube or windpipe is called the *trachea*. This starts just under the larynx and soon divides into two short tubes called the main *bronchi* ('bron-key') – one for each lung. The right bronchus is shorter than the left and more directly in line with the trachea.

The two bronchi enter the lungs and immediately branch into three smaller bronchi on the right side and two on the left. These continue to branch, and the branches lead to three lung lobes on the right side and two on the left. The lobes in turn are subdivided into a total of 19 separate lung segments, and the air passes into all of these.

The trachea and all the bronchi are supported and kept open by thin flexible rings, or partial rings, of gristle (*cartilage*), but as the size becomes less, these reinforcements are lost. The smaller, self-supporting air tubes are called *bronchioles* ('bron-key-oles'), which simply means 'small bronchi'. You probably don't appreciate how small and narrow the bronchioles really are. In fact, they are only about one millimetre in diameter – less than one sixteenth of an inch – and the smallest bronchi are not much bigger. This has important implications, as we shall see.

The inner lining of all the air tubes consists of a layer of rather remarkable cells. The free surfaces of these are covered with tiny, hair-like structures called *cilia* ('silly-ah'). These are essentially microscopic muscles that can bend in different directions. The extraordinary thing about them is that they all bend together in a purposeful way to produce a wafting motion, exactly like wind blowing across a field of ripe corn. Between the cilia are many hollow cells that manufacture mucus and squeeze it out onto the surface. These are called *goblet cells*. The cilia and the mucus work together to keep the air tubes clear. If the air breathed in contains any fine particles of foreign material, these are trapped by the mucus and are then carried upwards, by the mass action of the cilia, into the main bronchi and larynx. Once there, their presence causes us to cough and get rid of them. Recent research suggests that, in addition to all the other problems suffered by severe asthmatics, this important mechanism may, as we shall see, be disrupted.

The smallest bronchioles end in little expansions from which bud out the millions of tiny air sacs called the *alveoli* ('ahl-vee-ole-ee'). It is to these that the whole complicated system is dedicated, because it is in the alveoli that the breathed-in air comes into close contact with the blood. The walls of the alveoli are very thin indeed and they are wrapped round by the smallest and thinnest kind of blood vessels – the *capillaries*. Indeed, in places, the walls of the alveoli and the walls of the capillaries appear to be one and the same thing. So, with air in the alveoli and blood in the capillaries it is easy for oxygen to diffuse across into the blood, and for the waste gas carbon dioxide to diffuse out.

You will see that the lung system is like an inverted tree. Indeed, doctors often refer to it as the bronchial tree.

What happens during an asthma attack?

There is one more important thing to be said about the lung structure. All the air tubes, whether supported by cartilage or not, have muscle fibres in their walls. These are *involuntary* (smooth) muscles and we have no control over when and how they function. They run circularly in such a way that when they tighten they squeeze and narrow the tube. This is especially important in the smaller bronchi and in the bronchioles. If these muscles contract fully, the air tubes are closed off altogether and breathing is impossible. Fortunately, this very rarely occurs in all of the air tubes.

As you will now probably have guessed, asthma has much to do with the tightening of these muscles. In a severe attack, many of the smaller tubes can be closed off altogether and most of the others considerably narrowed. But it is not only the tightening of the muscles that narrows the airways. An asthmatic attack also features swelling of the lining cells of the tubes and overactivity of the goblet cells, so that far more mucus than normal is produced and the tubes further obstructed. The result is predictable – a rapid drop in the amount of air getting to the alveoli, wheezing, breathlessness, and often a cough with sputum production.

Ironically, these effects make it easier to breathe in than to breathe out. It is characteristic of an asthmatic attack that breathing out takes longer than breathing in, so air gets trapped in the lungs. The air soon loses its oxygen to the blood, and after that it is useless, simply taking up space in the lungs that you can ill afford. The extra difficulty in getting rid of the unwanted air means that the chest remains partly expanded and most of the exhausting effort is expended in trying actively to empty the lungs. Normally, this is a completely passive process that occurs as a result of the elasticity of the lungs, with no effort.

How does blood carry oxygen?

The blood contains millions of tiny saucer-shaped red cells. There are about five million of these in each cubic millimetre. Each red cell contains a protein and iron-containing substance called *haemoglobin* which has a remarkable ability to link with oxygen. When haemoglobin is in a situation where there is plenty of oxygen, it picks up a maximum load. But when it is in a low-oxygen area, it immediately gives up its linked oxygen. So when haemoglobin passes through the lungs it takes up oxygen, and when it reaches the cells of the body – which have an insatiable demand for oxygen – it gives it up. That's all there is to it. Because the heart keeps the blood circulating, first through the lungs and then through the body, there is a constant flow of oxygen from the air sacs in the lungs to the body cells everywhere.

The greatest requirement for oxygen is in the brain. So, in the main arteries carrying blood to the brain there are little monitors – groups of special cells called the carotid bodies – that keep a constant watch on the amount of oxygen in the blood. If this drops, a message is immediately sent to the part of the brain that controls breathing, prompting it to speed up and deepen the breathing. This automatic control works perfectly if the air tubes are wide open. Whenever we exert ourselves and use up oxygen more quickly, our rate and depth of breathing are immediately increased. And when we are at rest, the breathing remains quiet. But if the air tubes are narrowed and partly blocked so that less oxygen gets through the blood, the carotid bodies act at once to try to increase the breathing.

This is the dilemma facing the asthma sufferer who is having a severe attack. The factors that are causing the levels of oxygen in the blood to drop are also the factors that prevent the body from automatically correcting the trouble.

The nature of asthma

Just about the only good thing one can say about asthma is that, unlike other conditions that narrow the air tubes – conditions like chronic bronchitis, emphysema, cystic fibrosis or bronchiectasis – asthma doesn't cause trouble all the time. For someone with established asthma, the liability to attack is, of course, always there. But, for most sufferers, there are periods of days or weeks during which there is no way of proving that the people concerned *are* asthmatic. Surprisingly, there are no specific tests for asthma.

Another distinguishing feature is that the degree of obstruction to the airflow in the lungs can vary widely at different times. It can also change suddenly – in a matter of minutes – or gradually get worse, or better, over the course of days or weeks. Recovery from an attack may occur spontaneously or may be the result of treatment. All these features distinguish asthma from the other conditions.

The importance of inflammation

Recent research has emphasized that asthma is far more than simply a process that narrows the air tubes. Although this is the most striking and obvious feature of the disease, asthma is now regarded as essentially a disorder of the air tube linings involving persistent *inflammation*. Inflammation means widening and increased leakiness of blood vessels, causing local swelling, and an outpouring of cells of the immune system. The importance of the inflammatory element has been established by taking samples of the air tube linings and washings of the air tube secretions and examining them. Inflammation has been found to be present in even the mildest cases of asthma and in all cases the cells characteristic of inflammation are found to be present. In the great majority of cases this inflammation is allergic in origin. The inflammation inevitably adds to the narrowing of the air tubes.

Inflammation may be *acute* (short-lived) or *chronic* (tending to become permanent). It always starts as an acute condition, but if it is not checked at the acute stage it is all too liable to become chronic. Chronic inflammation means structural changes, such as scarring from fibrous tissue production and loss of the normal features of muscle and lining cells. These changes may become permanent, and it is thought to be because of them that many cases of asthma, once fully established, last for a lifetime.

A case in point is that of the industrial asthma caused by inhaling toluene di-isocyanate, a chemical used in the manufacture of polyurethane products. Many workers exposed to this compound rapidly develop asthma. If the cause is appreciated within about six months and exposure stopped, the asthma soon clears up and is cured. But if exposure continues for more than about six months, the asthma becomes permanent and continues even if the worker changes to an entirely different job.

This same process, in which an acute inflammation becomes chronic, may account for the fact that three-quarters of the cases of childhood asthma clear up completely in the teens, while a quarter become life-long problems. These new facts also have important implications for the treatment of early asthma and, as we shall see, the emphasis today is as much on the control of inflammation as on the relaxing of the tight muscles in the air tube walls.

Asthmatic attacks are triggered by a range of stimuli – some very common, some much less so (see below). These factors which bring on attacks can be divided into two large groups – the allergic triggers and the non-allergic stimuli. These distinct groups are so important that a whole chapter is devoted to each of them in this book.

Asthma starts more often in children under five than in any other age group. At that age, boys are affected up to twice as often as girls, but by the teens new cases occur as often in girls as in boys. By the age of about 20, the incidence of new cases has dropped to about half that of the peak occurring in young children. This decline in the number of new cases continues until it reaches a lowest point at about the age of 35 and then slowly rises again to about the age of 65.

Parents of young asthmatic children will be pleased to learn that a spontaneous cure is much commoner than is generally supposed. In fact, about a quarter of all affected children grow out of their asthma some time during adolescence and are not troubled thereafter. Those most likely to have this good fortune are children with comparatively infrequent attacks. Unfortunately, cures are much less common in adults and, regrettably, the tendency is for attacks to occur more often with the passage of time.

The incidence of asthma is about the same in Europe as in the USA. The figures reported for Australia and New Zealand are significantly higher, and those for Japan and North Canada, Alaska, Greenland and East Siberia are much lower. In Australia and New Zealand, the prevalence of asthma has recently been as high as 12 per cent in some groups of children. Inexplicably, the incidence in New Zealand is now falling. As we shall see, there are good reasons why asthma should be less comon in the frozen north and in alpine regions above about 1,000 metres. Perhaps surprisingly, the prevalence of asthma is also very low in most developing countries, especially in village communities.

Types of asthma

All types of asthma affect people in the same way. So far as the symptoms and effects on the life of the individual are concerned, asthma is asthma. But if one wishes to combat a disease, it is very important to know what causes it and what brings on attacks. So, in terms of causation, attempts have always been made to distinguish different types of asthma.

The distinction between these different types of asthma has probably been drawn too firmly in the past. Asthma used to be divided into *extrinsic* (allergic) asthma and *intrinsic* (non-allergic) asthma. Unfortunately, one cannot simply divide all cases into allergic asthma and non-allergic asthma, as the chapter headings of this book might seem to imply. There are lots of people who have a most obviously allergic type of asthma and know it. But there are also many people whose attacks are brought on by a variety of different trigger factors, some clearly connected with allergy, some not. Finally, there is a group of asthma sufferers with no history of allergic problems, no family history of allergy, negative skin tests for allergy and no indication on laboratory testing that there is any allergic element present. These people are said to have *idiopathic* asthma. This sounds impressive but the word idiopathic is just a medical buzz-word meaning 'I don't know the cause'.

These non-allergic cases are comparatively uncommon and it has to be said that, in the great majority of cases of asthma, there is an allergic element, sometimes minor, sometimes only too obvious. Allergy is the cause of asthma in 90 per cent of affected people below the age of 16. In older people, asthma is less often of allergic origin, but it is so in 70 per cent of people below the age of 30 and in 50 per cent of those over this age. This being so, it is very important for you to know as much as possible about allergy and its connection with asthma. That is what the next chapter is all about.

What starts an asthma attack?

Asthmatic attacks may be triggered by many different stimuli, but each individual sufferer tends to have his or her own particular triggers. The following list is not comprehensive, but includes the most important triggers for an attack:

- tree or grass pollens
- ragweed pollen (especially in the USA)
- fungal spores
- kapok and feather stuffing for pillows, etc.
- animal skin flakes (dander)
- house dust mite droppings
- hair particle proteins
- a few food additives, such as tartrazine
- changes in temperature or humidity
- strong smells
- fumes of various kinds
- atmospheric ozone
- smoke pollution
- atmospheric sulphur dioxide
- emotional upset
- stress
- colds and other upper respiratory tract infections
- discharge from the sinuses
- various drugs, especially beta-blockers and aspirin
- alcohol
- betel-nut chewing
- nuts
- shellfish
- some fruits

- strenuous exertion, especially in cold air
- reflux of acid into the lower gullet
- common colds.

While some of these obviously imply allergy, it is important to appreciate that *any* of these triggers may start an attack of asthma, whether or not the asthma is allergic in nature. Taking a beta-blocker drug, for instance, is liable to bring on an attack of asthma in *any* asthmatic person. The fact that the trigger that usually brings on an attack is clearly not connected with allergy – as in the case of triggers such as stress, emotional upset or severe exertion – does not imply that the asthma is not basically allergic in nature. These triggers *precipitate* the attack – they are not necessarily the underlying cause.

The symptoms of asthma

The most obvious symptoms, present in most cases, are:

- difficulty in breathing, especially in breathing out;
- wheezing, so that breathing becomes distinctly audible;
- cough;
- tightness of the chest;
- unduly rapid breathing;
- rapid heart rate.

The expiration difficulty quickly results in more breath being taken in than is expired. As a result, the chest becomes inflated and looks larger than normal. Doctors usually detect this by putting the fingers of one hand flat on the chest and briskly tapping the back of one of them with the middle finger of the other hand. This is called *percussion* and it produces a typically resonant sound. Breathing difficulty varies strikingly from time to time. Often it is so severe that it is impossible to do anything but fight for breath. Getting breath may be so difficult that it is quite impossible to remain lying down. Even if exhausted, the person simply has to sit up or stand and will often go to a window in the hope of getting more air. Some people will sit with their elbows on their knees.

Asthmatic wheezing produces a random series of sounds of different pitch, some quite musical in nature, which may occur at different phases of the expiration or inspiration. They occur, of course, only during an attack. A musical wheeze that is constantly present, and that does not vary in character, is not due to asthma but is caused by a fixed obstruction such as an inhaled foreign body or a tumour in a bronchus.

Typically, the cough of asthma is sometimes dry and sometimes produces large amounts of sputum. The cause of the sputum is explained later (see chapter 2). This sputum may be quite yellow, but it does not follow from this that infection is present. Certainly, pus usually implies infection, but in this case the cells that cause the yellowing are not the usual inflammatory cells of pus; they are cells called *eosinophils* present only in large numbers in allergic conditions and in worm infestations.

Chest tightness is an unpleasant sensation that may sometimes be severe enough to raise the suspicion of a heart attack or angina. It has, of course, nothing to do with the heart, but is the effect of being unable to take in a full and satisfying breath.

The increase in the rate of breathing occurs in spite of the breathing difficulty. The reason for this is that it has to. The necessity to get enough oxygen is so great that whenever the blood levels drop, the rate of breathing is automatically increased. This is exactly the same mechanism that causes us to breathe more rapidly when we exert ourselves. There would not be much point in breathing more rapidly if the blood passing through the lungs were already fully saturated with oxygen. But if the blood oxygen levels are low, then both an increased breathing rate and an increase in the rate at which blood passes through the lungs are valuable. So in addition to speeding up the breathing rate, the heart rate is also increased.

Now that you know how important allergy is in asthma, let's take a look at this mysterious entity – the allergic reaction.

2

Understanding allergic asthma

CASE HISTORY

When the Walpoles moved to a new house in the country their only child Jeremy seemed very happy at first. But within a few days things changed . . .

PERSONAL DETAILS

Name: Jeremy Walpole
Age: 7
Occupation: Schoolboy
Family: No siblings. Parents alive and well.

THE PRESENT COMPLAINT

Recently the parents moved to this area from London. After less than a week in the new house Jeremy began to cough and wheeze. Occasionally he has seemed quite distressed. He was due to start a new school but this has been postponed. His father tells the doctor that even just a game of chasing after him and tickling him can bring on a severe wheeze. The parents confirm that there are many trees and grasses in the vicinity of their new house.

MEDICAL BACKGROUND

The doctor asks about Jeremy's previous medical history. Jeremy's mother says that he was a healthy full-term, 8-pound baby. His medical history is unremarkable except for a moderately severe eczema that started when he was about nine months old. This affected the creases behind his knees and at his elbows, and later spread to his trunk. There was severe itching and constant scratching, but the trouble was finally brought under control with skin oil and a mild steroid cream. The eczema seemed to clear up altogether when he was five.

THE FAMILY HISTORY

Both parents are healthy but Jeremy's father thinks he had a tendency to bronchitis as a child. Jeremy's mother says that her mother, now deceased, was a martyr to hay fever.

THE EXAMINATION

The doctor notes that Jeremy is tall for his age and well nourished. The skin is clear with no sign of scaly patches or inflammation (dermatitis). There is a hint of indrawing of the chest on either side just below the nipples. Possibly the chest is rather more fully inflated than normal. This is confirmed when the doctor taps (*percusses*) Jeremy's chest and notes that the sound is more resonant than usual. After asking Jeremy to breathe in and out deeply and rapidly the doctor listens to his chest with a stethoscope. He tells the parents that there are some prolonged whistles – he calls them *ronchi* – on expiration.

The doctor shows Jeremy a tubular instrument with a dial and asks him to see how far up the scale he can move the needle by blowing into it as hard as he can. He shows him how. He checks the result on each of several tries, encouraging Jeremy to do better each time. He explains that this is a peak flow meter and that the test shows that Jeremy's ability to breathe out is below normal.

THE DIAGNOSIS

To the parents' surprise, the doctor seems especially interested in Jeremy's eczema and in his grandmother's hay fever. He also asks about the variety of trees near the Walpoles' home. Finally he announces that Jeremy has allergic asthma. He explains that the condition is mild and that, in view of the time of year – mid-April – it is probably brought on by tree pollen, possibly Birch.

Jeremy's father knows very little about asthma and is not particularly perturbed. 'But what has all this to do with the eczema?' he asks. 'Is there any connection?'

'Certainly,' says the doctor. 'It has a great deal to do with his eczema. And with his grandmother. And, incidentally, with his immune system.'

You, too, may be puzzled by the connection between asthma, eczema, grandmother's hay fever and the immune system. But read on and all will be explained.

The nature of allergy

Allergy is an excessive sensitivity – a *hypersensitivity* – to a particular substance that comes in contact with some part of the body. Any substance that causes allergy is called an *allergen*. There are plenty of these, but different groups of allergens tend to cause different types of allergy. Skin contact allergies cause hives or nettle-rash (*urticaria*) or dermatitis; food allergies – which are rare – cause tummy upsets; and grass or tree pollen allergies or dust mite dropping allergies cause asthma or hay fever. The allergic reaction, whatever it is, never occurs on the first contact with the allergen, but only on repeated contact. Between the first and later contacts a great deal goes on in the body's immune system.

How the immune system is involved

Allergy is a disorder of the immune system. Most people are familiar with what happens when the immune system fails to act properly, as in AIDS. Allergy is at the opposite end of the spectrum of immune disorders and is really what happens when the immune system acts all too vigorously. The system is, of course, dedicated to protecting us from foreign invaders, especially viruses, bacteria, fungi and so on. It does this by manufacturing special proteins called *antibodies* or *immunoglobulins* which latch on to the invaders, mark them, and immobilize them so that the eating and scavenging cells of the system (the *phagocytes*) can destroy them. The immune system doesn't, of course, know whether any tiny item of foreign material is dangerous or not. It just knows that it is different from its own substances. All of our own body cells carry identifying markers – small chemical groups on their surfaces – which tell the immune system cells that they are 'self' and should be left alone. But when foreign cells or large chemical groups get into the body these ID cards are missing, or different, and the immune system knows to attack them.

Antibodies are made by a class of cells known as B lymphocytes – B cells for short – and they do an excellent job of protection. There are thousands of different kinds of antibodies, each one exactly right (*specific*) to tackle a particular foreign invader. Remember that they are soluble *globulin* proteins. Antibodies are called *immunoglobulins*. There are five classes of antibodies, and in allergy we are particularly concerned with one of the classes – the immunoglobulin class E. This is really too much of a mouthful, so doctors talk about IgE. Ig is short for immunoglobulin. Most people with allergic asthma have more IgE than other people.

The mast cells

In addition to the B cells and the phagocytes, the immune system uses many other kinds of cells. Among these are a group of special interest in allergy called the *mast cells*. These occur in large numbers all over the body. They are especially prevalent in the air tubes of asthma sufferers. Some are in the walls, just under the lining; others are free inside the tubes, on the surface of the lining. Mast cells are white cells which, when stained and examined under the micro-scope, are seen to contain large numbers of granules that stain deeply. They were first noted by the celebrated German bacteriologist and discoverer of the first real cure for syphilis, Paul Ehrlich (1854–1915). Ehrlich thought the granules were material that the cells had eaten, and since *mast* is German for pig food, that is what he called them.

Chemical microanalysis shows that the mast cell granules consist of a cocktail of powerful and unpleasant substances most of which cause severe inflammation when they come in contact with other body cells. These substances include histamine, leukotrienes and prostaglandins, all of which are well-known body irritants. Hay fever sufferers will be familiar with histamine, because their principal remedy is one of the large range of antihistamine drugs. Histamine and the leukotrienes are powerful trigger substances that tighten the muscles in the walls of the air tubes (bronchi and bronchioles – see chapter 1). Prostaglandins are released from any kind of cell that is injured, and are the cause of the associated pain. They are also used to cause abortion.

All things considered, these granules are best left safely alone within the mast cells. Unfortunately for people with allergic asthma, the IgE has other ideas. Mast cells have on their surface particular locking-on bays (*receptor sites*) that fit exactly with IgE. As a result, when the immune system makes IgE proteins – and each B cell can do so at a rate of 2,000 per second – these soon find themselves firmly latched on to the mast cells. There is no harm in this. But remember that the IgE is specially selected to deal with a particular foreign substance and will always, if it can, attach itself to that substance. Let us assume that, in this case, the substance is a few particles of house mite droppings inhaled when bedsheets are shaken. These droppings are coated with the enzymes the mites use to digest the skin scales on which they live, and it is the enzymes that are the real allergens. So, naturally, the allergen particles latch on to the IgE that is already fixed to the mast cells.

How mast cells degranulate

All over the surface of each mast cell are many IgE molecules. Whenever a mite dropping enzyme links to two adjacent IgE antibodies a strain is applied to the mast cell membrane. It requires very few allergens – perhaps only one – to strain the cell membrane so much that it tears. When it does, of course, the granules are released. Doctors use the impressive term *degranulation*, but this is all it means. The mast cell outer cover is torn, and histamine, leukotrienes, prostaglandins and other nasty substances are let out.

This is where the hypersensitivity comes from. These mite allergens, like pollen grains, are microscopic, but their effect as triggers can be devastating. Granule substances released from mast cells immediately act on the air tubes. They do so in four ways:

- they cause the circularly placed muscles in the walls of the tubes to tighten and so narrow the tubes;
- they cause small blood vessels in the walls to widen so that the walls are thickened;
- they cause these vessels to leak more fluid so that the walls become waterlogged and further thickened;
- they cause the goblet cell glands in the tube linings to produce more muscus.

All these effects lead to a striking reduction in the ability of air to get through the tubes. The smaller bronchioles can be closed off altogether and the effect on the person concerned can be terrifying. There is danger that he or she may be deprived of the element literally most vital to life – oxygen.

What is the point of having mast cells?

Since degranulation of mast cells appears to be exclusively against our personal interest, this question has worried immunologists ever since the function of the mast cells was discovered. In the course of evolution, the changes that give rise to new body constituents do not succeed unless there is some good reason. A clue to the possible reasons for our having mast cells is the fact that in two conditions they are commonly accompanied by other similar-looking and granule-containing cells called *eosinophils*. The two conditions in which eosinophils are common are allergies and worm infestations.

Worms stimulate the production of IgE and this causes mast cells to release their granules in the vicinity of the worms. We now know that among the substances released from the granules is a factor that strongly attracts eosinophils to the site. The eosinophils then attack the worms, crowding round them and attracting to them antibodies that damage them. The worms are then coated with mucus and are unable to resist being expelled from the gut.

During the course of evolution all humans, and the primates from which we evolved, had worms, and it seems likely that the mast cells developed to help to get rid of them. But now that we have done even better than nature, and produced highly effective drugs to dispose of worms, it is likely that we could happily do without the mast cells. Regrettably, at least for the foreseeable future, we are stuck with them.

Why do some people have allergies while others do not?

People with allergic asthma usually have a family history of certain conditions grouped under the term *atopy*. These conditions are asthma, hay fever (*allergic rhinitis*) and eczema (*allergic dermatitis*). A diagnosis of atopy can also be suggested by various laboratory tests, including tests for increased numbers of mast cells, tests for levels of IgE in the blood, skin tests to various allergens, and tests that identify the specific kinds of IgE for particular allergens.

Although atopy can show itself in these distinct ways, it does tend to follow one particular pattern in families. In some families with atopy, all or most of the affected members have hay fever; in others all or most will have asthma; in yet others, eczema will be the feature. We also know that atopic disease, however it presents, is more commonly inherited from the mother than from the father.

Since atopy runs very strongly in families it is obviously genetic in origin, although, of course, there are also major environmental factors in any allergic condition. In the light of what you now know, you could define atopy as a state in which excessive production of IgE usually occurs as a response to contact with environmental allergens. We have to say 'usually' because some people with atopic eczema have normal levels of IgE. In recent years there have been many important advances in our understanding of asthma; among the most important of these is new knowledge of the genetic basis of the condition. It has long been assumed that there must be a genetic basis to asthma, and there are all kinds of reasons for thinking so. One impressive illustration of this is the situation on the isolated volcanic island of Tristan da Cunha, where, of the 15 original settlers, three women were asthmatic. Today, over 30 per cent of the population suffer from asthma. Most of the sufferers are female.

The genetic link

Quite recently, the chromosome that carries the abnormal gene for the atopic tendency to allergic problems has been identified by a group of British and Japanese scientists working in Oxford, led by Julian Hopkins of the Churchill Hospital. This group began to study the genetic link with asthma in 1985, working on DNA samples from 100 families with atopy. By 1989 they had narrowed down the search to chromosome number 11, and by August 1991 had established that a particular section of chromosome 11 was implicated.

This gene variant is very common: 85 per cent of those carrying the gene have some kind of symptoms, 60 per cent have wheeze and 20 per cent have asthma. Inheritance of this gene has been found to occur only through the female line. This presents a problem as we already know that atopy can, although less commonly, be inherited from the father. The researchers, however, are fairly certain that the gene they have isolated is responsible for only about 60 per cent of cases of atopy. It must be presumed that there is at least one other gene for paternally transmitted atopy. The experts believe that half a dozen different genes and many environmental factors are involved in the production of atopy.

The abnormal gene on chromosone 11 is actually responsible for producing an abnormal receptor on the surface of mast cells – a receptor to which IgE attaches itself, as we have seen. Surprisingly, the rogue gene is only very slightly different from the normal one, and the protein receptor formed by it differs from the normal receptor by only one amino acid. Amino acids are the 'building bricks' which are strung together in a particular order to produce proteins. The properties of proteins are critically dependent on the right amino acids being present in the right order. Even so, this difference is tiny, but it is enough to make the IgE receptor far more sensitive than usual, so that the mast cells disintegrate more easily. So here, at last, is an explanation that provides the known facts of atopic asthma with a clear genetic basis.

Evidence from lung transplantation

Some evidence has come to light that helps to show where the genetic factors operate. It was reported in May 1993 that when lungs from donors who were asthmatic are transplanted into patients who are not asthmatic, the recipients develop asthma. And when lungs from non-asthmatics are transplanted into people with severe asthma, the disease is cured. This unique evidence is of great interest. It indicates that, in addition to the immunological changes described above – which affect the whole body – there are specific changes, or differences, in the lungs of people with asthma.

3
The other forms of asthma

CASE HISTORY

Gerry has always prided himself on his fitness and good health. Until, quite suddenly, at the age of 27, he began to have disabling attacks of breathlessness.

PERSONAL DETAILS

Name: Gerry Forsythe
Age: 27
Occupation: Solicitor's clerk
Family: Two sisters. No health problems. Both parents alive and well.

MEDICAL BACKGROUND

This is unremarkable. Gerry had the usual minor childhood illnesses, including mumps and chickenpox, but has had no major illnesses or injuries. He is a keen amateur football player and has been accustomed to vigorous weekly training sessions and a match every Saturday during the season. He is happy in his work and enjoys his hobby of electronic equipment construction.

THE PRESENT COMPLAINT

Gerry reports to his GP complaining that for about two months he has been having alarming attacks of breathlessness. He has also noticed that, in spite of keeping up his training, he seems to be much less fit than he used to be. In several games he has lost opportunities because he simply has not had the stamina needed. He gets breathless much more easily than he did earlier in the season.

THE HISTORY AND EXAMINATION

The doctor asks many questions and seems to be especially interested in any suggestion of chest pain or discomfort on exertion. Gerry confirms that there has been no such symptom. To Gerry's surprise, the doctor asks about his parents' health. So far as he is aware, neither of them have ever had any significant illnesses. The doctor persists, enquiring whether there is any question of heart trouble on either side of the family. Gerry is sure there has been nothing of that kind.

Gerry is then asked to strip to the waist. His chest is examined carefully by inspection, a check of breathing movements, percussion and listening all over with the stethoscope. The doctor then runs an electrocardiogram.

When he is finished, the doctor tells Gerry that he has been able to find nothing wrong with either the heart or the lungs and is unable to account for the attacks and the loss of fitness. He suggests a referral to a hospital consultant.

THE HOSPITAL OUT-PATIENT CHECK

The consultant asks all the same questions as the GP and repeats the examination. He assures Gerry that his heart is normal, but then branches out into a wider area. Does he, or either of his parents, have hay fever or asthma or skin trouble? What are conditions like at his work? What has changed in his life-style over the period during which he has been having the attacks? Gerry gives negative answers to all these questions, but the consultant persists. What about his spare-time activities? Any new hobbies?

Gerry laughs and says that the only change is that he recently began to take an interest in electronic construction. He has assembled a complete HI-FI from a series of kits and is very pleased with the results. The consultant shows a surprising degree of interest. 'Printed-circuit boards?' he asks. 'Integrated circuits? Resistors and capacitors? Soldering?'

'Of course', says Gerry.

'Rosin-cored solder?'

'Certainly.'

'Think carefully,' says the consultant, 'did the first attack occur before or after you took up this hobby?'

'Oh, after. I started working on the projects four or five months ago.'

'So it was soldering first and attacks after?'

Gerry's eyes widen. 'The smoke from the solder . . .' he says. 'Of course . . . I've been breathing it in. You have to get really close to make sure you don't short these tiny pins. Could that possibly . . .?'

The consultant tells him that inhaling colophony flux vapour is a well-recognized cause of asthma.

THE FOLLOW-UP

A little experimentation shows that this is indeed the cause of Gerry's breathlessness. Within a few hours of inhaling the vapour from rosin-cored electronic wire solder he invariably has an acute attack. Within two months, his performance on the football field has returned to normal. Gerry is now putting together a personal computer – a job that requires no soldering.

The environment and asthma

There is increasing evidence that one of the reasons for the steady rise in the incidence of asthma – possibly the main reason – is the rise in atmospheric pollution, especially in cities. There are two main sources of pollution: industrial effluent and heavy concentrations of motor vehicles. The latter is often the most obvious. The East London Borough of Tower Hamlets is a case in point. Children in this area are exposed to high levels of atmospheric pollution and the admission rate for asthma to the local hospital is 80 per cent above the national average. The pollution is mainly from motor vehicles but domestic smoking may also be a factor.

In a response to this situation, a research project was started in September 1994, in which 100 children from primary schools in the borough will use peak flow meters, morning and evening, and record the results. Some of them will also carry monitor badges that detect and measure levels of atmospheric chemical pollution. The Tower Hamlets experience is by no means unique. In inner-city areas generally children and others are being exposed to alarmingly high levels of vehicular pollution.

The reason why these pollutants affect the prevalence of asthma is gradually becoming clear. Many of them, especially the nitrogen oxides from car exhausts and the ozone that is produced when sunlight acts on these oxides, are damaging to the ciliated lining of the air tubes (see chapter 1). These remarkable cells, with their 'brush border' of moving hairs, are, when healthy, highly effective in carrying fine particles and mucus out of the respiratory system. Among these particles are the allergens (see chapter 2) which cause the asthmatic attack.

We now know that nitrogen oxides, even in quite low concentrations, can damage the cilia-bearing cells: 0.4 parts per million of nitrogen dioxide, for instance, will interfere with the action of the cilia. Two parts per million will kill the cilia cells. If this happens, the allergens, whatever they may be, are obviously going to be kept longer in contact with the small air tubes, so that they are more likely to trigger an allergic response. The levels of these dangerous oxides from traffic fumes have been rising steadily for years and have been accompanied by a similar rise in the number and severity of cases of asthma. This association also helps to explain the surprising fact that asthma, like hay fever, is commoner in towns than in the country, in spite of the fact that pollen sources are more plentiful in rural setting.

The association between ozone and allergic asthma has also been investigated. The *Lancet* of 27 July 1991 carries a leading article from Toronto about a deliberate trial of the effects of very low concentrations of inhaled ozone on the tendency to develop an asthmatic attack in allergic people. The concentration used in the trial was very low – only 0.12 parts per million in the inspired air. This concentration is similar to what occurs in any city area in which the traffic is heavy. The results were very definite. Inhalation of the ozone by itself did not affect the ability to breathe out forcibly. Inhalation of low concentrations of pollen allergen by itself likewise had no effect. But when inhalation of the allergen was followed by inhalation of the dilute ozone, there was a very obvious tightening of the air tubes with a reduction in the ability to blow out forcibly. The presence of the ozone reduced by half the dose of allergen needed to produce the allergic reaction.

The ozone concentrations in the atmosphere of some North American cities at the time of the trial were:

Los Angeles	0.33 parts per million
New York	0.18 parts per million
Baltimore	0.19 parts per million
Philadelphia	0.20 parts per million
Washington	0.18 parts per million
Chicago	0.22 parts per million
Houston	0.22 parts per million

Note that all these levels are well above the levels used in this study.

Industrial smoke effluents are also a source of nitrogen oxides but, in addition, they pump out into the atmosphere millions of tonnes of the irritating and dangerous gas sulphur dioxide. This is the gas that is mainly responsible for producing the acid rain that is so damaging to architecture and to trees. But sulphur dioxide is also damaging to human lungs. Very low concentrations will induce asthma. The compound is used as a preservative in wines and other beverages, and it has, for instance, been shown that an asthmatic attack can be brought on by inhaling the tiny amount released from the surface of wine in a glass in the course of drinking.

Allergy and occupation

Many substances encountered in an occupational situation – well over 200 – have been found capable of precipitating an asthmatic attack. In the industrial environment, the worker may be exposed to far higher concentrations of these substances than are the consumers. Also, industrial processes often involve release into the atmosphere of fine dusts arising from the offending substances.

Most of these substances fall into groups, but some individual materials are especially liable to cause trouble. The commonest industrial asthma-promoting agents are:

- platinum salts
- isocyanates
- colophony resins in solder
- weevil-infested wheat flour
- *Penicillium* spores from mouldy cheese
- mushroom compost
- green coffee beans
- soya bean dust
- tea powder
- tobacco powder
- cork dust
- wood pulp
- hairdressing chemicals such as ammonium persulphate
- various drugs in powder form
- silk
- cotton
- dyes
- plants
- various sawdusts and wood dusts, especially oak, boxwood and cedar
- vegetable dusts, such as castor bean and coffee bean
- natural gums (tragacanth, gum arabic and gum acacia)
- protein-splitting and other biological enzymes

- drugs, especially antibiotics, cimetidine and piperazine
- trimellitic and other anhydrides (epoxy resin curing agents)
- metal salts, especially platinum, nickel and chrome
- vapour from soldering and brazing fluxes (colophony fumes)
- animal products, especially urine
- irritant gases
- formaldehyde
- environmental smokes
- paints
- solvents
- PVC
- gum acacia
- salts of chromium, nickel, cobalt and vanadium.

Some of these substances are more liable to bring on asthma than others. Bakers' flour has been known to cause asthma since ancient times. It is a potent allergen. Not only can the flour itself cause allergies, but it often contains other allergens such as mites, fungal spores and finely chopped wheat hairs. Some 20 per cent of bakers exposed to wheat flour develop asthma.

Platinum salt dusts will cause asthma in as many as 50 per cent of workers exposed to them and there are stringent regulations governing the working conditions of those who might be exposed to them. Any who reveal sensitivity to platinum by skin prick testing are excluded from such employment. About the same proportion of workers who are exposed to protein-splitting enzymes develop asthma.

About 10 per cent of people working with toluene di-isocyanate develop asthma. The isocyanates are used in the manufacture of polyurethane foams, paints and wire and electronic component insulation. Asthma is also common in workers exposed to the dust of Canadian red cedar wood, South African boxwood, oak and Mansonia woods. About one in 20 workers exposed to these dusts develop asthma. The allergen, in these cases, is plicatic acid in the wood.

Trimellitic anhydride (TMA) and phthalic acid anhydride are hardening agents used to set epoxy resins. They are also used as plasticizers. They are potent allergens. Once specific IgE levels to these have built up following initial exposure, a reaction – such as an asthma attack – will be apparent within minutes of further exposure. These allergens can also produce other unpleasant effects such as hay fever, muscle pains, coughing of blood, high temperature and anaemia.

The term 'industrial' should not, in this context, be limited to the professional workplace; many of these substances can arise in the course of hobbies and leisure-time activities. In this case, because the conditions are not subject to industrial safety regulations, and because safety precautions are often ignored, the risk may actually be greater than during paid activities.

Most cases of occupational asthma disappear when the person concerned is no longer exposed to the particular substance, either by better working conditions with more effective protection, or by a change of job. Regrettably, there are some cases in which asthma induced in this way becomes permanent. The history of industrial asthma is often quite typical. Here is a case study that illustrates this point:

CASE HISTORY

Kirsty works in a small chromium plating plant concerned mainly with replating parts such as bumpers and bonnets for vintage cars. She has not been long at this occupation when she realizes that all is not as it should be.

PERSONAL DETAILS

Name: Kirsty Sandburg
Age: 33
Occupation: Electroplating technician
Family: Single. Parents dead. No siblings.

MEDICAL BACKGROUND

Kirsty had a chest problem as a child and was said to have chronic bronchitis. This seemed to clear, however, and by her early 20s she seemed healthy enough. She is a heavy cigarette smoker and seldom takes exercise. She is rather overweight. She has had many jobs and took up her present occupation about five months ago.

THE PRESENT COMPLAINT

Kirsty takes a day off to visit her doctor. Her complaint is that nearly every day she develops quite a severe cough, tightness in her chest and some difficulty in breathing.

THE HISTORY

The doctor takes a history of the complaint and discovers at once that the trouble occurs only when she is at work. She is always quite all right on arriving for work but towards the end of the shift the symptoms develop. They continue to get worse for a time after the shift, but then settle down. The doctor asks her about weekends and holidays, and it becomes clear that she is never then affected. The doctor asks what her work involves and she explains that she is concerned with a late stage of the process – clamping on the electric contacts and lowering the articles into the plating bath of chromium salt solution.

'Are there any suction fans over the vats?'

'No. Nothing like that. Or at least there are fans but they're never turned on. Too noisy. You can't hear the music.'

He asks whether anyone else in the firm has similar trouble.

'Oh, yes', says Kirsty. 'They nearly all get it. It's called platers' cough. Best thing for it is to keep a cig going.'

THE DOCTOR'S COMMENTS

The doctor soon disabuses her of this idea. After examining her chest and finding no abnormal signs, he explains that the problem is due to inhaling vapour from the chromic acid in the plating bath. This, he says, is a frequent cause of asthma. He explains that if she goes on having the trouble too long, there is a real chance that it might become permanent. He advises her to give up her job.

THE FOLLOW-UP

Kirsty had no intention of giving up her job. She finds the company at work very much to her taste and ignores the doctor's advice.

Her conscientious GP, however, submits a formal report on the case to the Health and Safety Executive and the premises of Kirsty's firm receive an unwelcome inspection. It appears that hardly any of the regulations are being complied with. The proprietors are duly warned that the business will be closed down unless they mend their ways. Kirsty continues to smoke as much as she can but is at least protected from the chromium, and she and her workmates have no further attacks of asthma.

Exercise and asthma

All exercise worthy of the name causes breathlessness, but this soon settles on resting. With asthma, however, the situation is different. Nearly all asthmatics know that an attack can be brought on by exertion, or that if an attack has started it can be made worse by exercise. This effect is most marked in cold dry conditions. What is not generally appreciated, however, is that, in some cases, exercise is the only thing that does bring on an attack. This is an important fact because experience shows that people in this category usually do not appreciate that they are suffering from asthma. Many of them simply imagine that they are 'unfit'. Unfortunately, such people often eventually develop asthma that occurs independently of exercise. People who wheeze on exertion should therefore be aware of this risk and should not dismiss the problem lightly. Everyone who experiences this effect should consult a doctor.

Asthmatics are also usually aware that an attack can readily be brought on by a change of atmospheric temperature. This is what happens in the air tubes when exercise is taken. Evaporation of water takes heat from the surroundings. As the inspired air is heated up to body temperature and is humidified from the fluid on the inner surfaces of the air tubes, it takes heat from the walls. The colder and drier the inspired air, and the higher the rate of air flow, the greater is the cooling effect. Air flow rate is, of course, much increased by exertion.

It is not entirely clear why cooling of the air tube walls causes an asthmatic attack, but it seems probable that it is connected with the widening of the blood vessels in the walls that is necessary to bring about re-warming after cooling.

In the light of all this it is possible to discover which sports are least likely to bring on an attack. Clearly, winter sports such as skiing, vigorous skating and ice hockey are not a particularly good idea for an asthmatic person. By contrast, however, swimming exercise is strongly recommended for the maintenance of fitness in asthmatic people. Such an activity involves breathing air which is already warmed and thoroughly moistened so that no cooling of the air passages is involved. There is just one proviso. A few people develop sensitivity to the chlorine used to sterilize swimming pool water so that any exposure to it is liable to provoke an attack.

So far as outdoor sports are concerned, those involving sustained exertion such as football and medium- and long-distance running are less suitable than those involving short bursts of exertion such as jumping, throwing and cricket. There are many 100-metre sprinters who put up an excellent performance in spite of being asthmatic. This is because it is unnecessary to breathe during the 10 seconds or so of the race. Exercise is so important for children that they should never be deprived of it simply on account of their asthma. Proper medication by inhaler (see chapters 7 and 8) should allow almost any child to enjoy, and benefit from, most forms of exercise.

Infections and asthma

Infections of the respiratory system, such as colds and influenza, are the commonest reasons for an acute worsening of asthma. Research shows that virus infections, rather than the kind of bacterial infections that cause tonsillitis, are mainly responsible. The mere presence of the viruses is insufficient to trigger attacks. It is the actual virus infection, with obvious symptoms such as fever, sore throat, cough, runny nose and aches and pains, that is liable to bring on a severe attack. The effect of these infections is quite persistent. Even after the virus infection has cleared up, the person concerned may be significantly more liable to severe asthmatic attacks for a period of two to eight weeks.

Every effort should be made, therefore, to avoid such infections. Influenza vaccination should be considered. Remember that colds are passed on as much by hand contact as by coughs and sneezes. The hands of a person with a cold are always heavily contaminated with viruses and everything he or she touches will also be contaminated. If you have to shake hands with someone with a cold, keep your fingers away from your nose or eyes until you have been able to wash your hands thoroughly. Viruses gain access to the body via the nose lining and the conjuctival membrane that covers the eyeballs and lines the eyelids. Colds are, quite literally, contagious.

Stress and asthma

There is no reason to believe that stress and the emotional reaction to it can actually cause a non-asthmatic person to develop asthma. But, equally, there is no doubt that emotional stress is a potent factor in affecting the severity of asthma. Severe asthma is also a misfortune that, in itself, evokes a strong emotional reaction.

Indeed, the emotional dimension is so important in asthma that an entire chapter is devoted to it (see chapter 9).

Aspirin and asthma

About 3 per cent of adult asthmatics are sensitive to aspirin. In these people, the tiniest dose of aspirin will induce a severe asthmatic attack. Aspirin-induced asthma seems to affect people with late-onset asthma more often than those who develop the disease in childhood. Many of them have nasal polyps.

Aspirin is by no means the only painkilling drug to induce asthma. If you suspect that you might have this problem, watch out for:

- indomethacin (Indocid)
- phenylbutazone (Butacote)
- fenoprofen (Fenopron)
- ibuprofen (Brufen)
- diclofenac (Voltarol)
- naproxen (Naprosyn)
- mefenamic acid (Ponstan)
- paracetamol (Panadol).

With the exception of the latter, you will probably know these drugs under the trade names, which are different from the generic names. A common trade name is given for each in brackets, but there are many other brand names. If you look on the packet you will find the generic names and will be able to identify the drug (see also chapter 11).

Asthma and pregnancy

Many women with asthma worry about pregnancy. This is partly because of incomplete information about the hereditary aspects of asthma and partly because of concern that pregnancy might make the asthma worse. As you will have learned from chapter 2, the tendency to allergic asthma – atopy – can certainly be inherited. But if there is a strong atopic strain in your family, you will almost certainly already be aware of this and will know what it implies. If you are atopic, you may well pass it on to your baby. In the present state of knowledge, the gene for atopy seems to come from the mother rather than from the father, so it is your family rather than your partner's that counts. But even if you do pass on the gene to your baby, there is only a 20-per-cent chance that he or she will develop asthma.

So far as the pregnancy is concerned, there is no particular reason to be concerned. The chances are that you will go through it without any trouble attributable to your asthma. In a large series of pregnant asthmatic women, 33 per cent found that their asthma was completely unaffected by the pregnancy, 33 per cent actually had significantly *less* trouble than usual, and 33 per cent found that their asthma was worse. If you find you are in the unlucky third, you will simply have to take a little more trouble with your normal asthma management. There is no reason to expect that your baby will be harmed.

You will know by the end of the third month how things are going to go during your pregnancy. Experience shows that the pattern shown in the first trimester is almost always followed throughout. Moreover, the same pattern will be repeated in subsequent pregnancies.

Although the treatment of asthma in pregnancy is the same as at any other time, you should be careful in the early weeks to take no more medication than is strictly necessary. You should also watch out for any favourite combination remedy that contains drugs other than the standard asthma medication. Certain drugs, that are sometimes used as adjuncts in the treatment of asthma, should be avoided altogether. These are:

- phenylpropanolamine
- phenylephrine
- adrenaline (except when given by a doctor)
- codeine
- potassium iodide
- phenobarbitone and other barbiturates
- tetracycline
- sulphonamides
- trimethoprim
- ciprofloxacin
- aminoglycoside antibiotics.

Check the labels of your medication for any of these names and if you find them, discuss the matter with your doctor. If antibiotics are needed, a penicillin or an erythromycin are safer than a tetracycline (achromycin, aureomycin, terramycin, tetracyn, doxycycline, minocycline etc.) or an aminoglycoside (amikacin, gentamycin, kanamycin, neomycin, netilmicin, tobramycin etc.) Tetracyclines can damage fetal liver, cause yellow discoloration of teeth and interfere with the growth of bones. Aminoglycosides can damage the inner ears and cause permanent impairment of hearing.

Asthma and sinusitis

There is a well-recognized association between sinusitis and asthma. Sinusitis is also commonly related to nasal polyps and these, too, are often present in people with asthma. Clinical studies have shown that if sinusitis in people with asthma is properly treated, by surgery if necessary, the great majority of those concerned will claim that their asthma is substantially improved. In one series, 15 out of 18 patients were able to reduce their steroid usage by 95 per cent. It seems that the more severe the sinusitis, the more difficult it is to treat the asthma.

The moral of this is that if there is any question of sinusitis or nasal polyps in your case, you need a consultation with an ear, nose and throat specialist with a view to checking whether you need treatment. So far as nasal polyps are concerned, the important condition is called *eosinophilic vasomotor rhinitis*. You can suspect this if your asthma is associated with a tendency to watery running of the nose, nasal stuffiness, sneezing and sometimes irritation and watering of the eyes.

Heartburn and asthma

This may seem an unlikely combination but, in fact, the two conditions occur in a considerable proportion of asthmatic people. When doctors checked the association between asthma and the underlying cause of heartburn – the abnormal movement of stomach acid up into the gullet (acid regurgitation) – the figures were even more impressive. Studies have shown that 45 to 65 per cent of people with asthma, both children and adults, have acid regurgitation. It seems that in a proportion of cases, acid reflux occurs without actually producing heartburn and that this makes their asthma worse. Asthma can even be induced by dripping acid into the lower end of the gullet through a tube.

Research has shown that the strongest association is between acid regurgitation and night-time asthmatic attacks with coughing and wheezing. This is not surprising, as acid reflux is encouraged by lying down. Bending over or straining can also precipitate an asthmatic attack. Remember that the gullet runs down through the centre of the chest very close to the windpipe and the lungs. Clinical experience has shown that if acid reflux in an asthmatic person is effectively treated, the asthma often improves.

4

Asthma in childhood

This chapter is not intended to be read in isolation. Most of what is contained in the rest of the book also applies to children, and it is of the greatest importance that anyone dealing with an asthmatic child should be aware of the principles underlying the causation and management of asthma.

From the point of view of symptoms, asthma in childhood is just the same as asthma occurring later in life. But, for several reasons, it is necessary to look especially closely at childhood asthma. For a start, asthma is remarkably common in children – the latest government figures show that in Britain one child in seven suffers from it. Asthma in children is also becoming steadily commoner because of atmospheric pollution and other factors. Moreover, many parents regard asthma in children as 'just a bit of a wheeze' and not as something that can quickly become potentially very serious. This view can be dangerously complacent. But, perhaps above all, children with asthma are defenceless and are critically dependent on their parents for relief of their suffering, and sometimes even for the saving of their lives. Nearly all the children who die from asthma do so because their parents – and, regrettably, sometimes their doctors – are unaware of the potential dangers and fail to take decisive action early enough.

CASE HISTORY

Petra is an asthmatic but has never been greatly troubled by it. The doctor is fairly sure that she is allergic to something in the household – probably animal dandruff – but Petra loves her two cats and her dog and can't bear to part with them. One day, matters take a turn for the worse.

PERSONAL DETAILS

Name: Petra Greenwald

Age: 7

Occupation: Schoolgirl

Family: Parents alive and well. Two brothers in good health.

MEDICAL BACKGROUND

Almost from birth, Petra has had a tendency to eczema. This greatly distressed her mother who spent a lot of money on dermatological advice and treatment. Petra had her first asthma attack when she was just two years old and has since had many episodes. The asthma comes on without any obvious cause, and she is convinced that it has nothing to do with the animals. None of her attacks have been severe enough to cause particular concern.

THE FAMILY HISTORY

Petra's mother is quite familiar with her troubles as there is a well-marked family history of eczema, hay fever and asthma on her side, affecting two of Petra's aunts. She is not too worried, however, as, in the case of both her sisters, the trouble cleared up completely by early adult life. Both Mrs Greenwald and her husband are heavy smokers.

At the age of seven Petra has her most severe attack to date.

THE FIRST SEVERE ATTACK

One day Petra complains of tightness in her chest. She begins to cough and to wheeze. She is constantly using her inhaler but apparently with little effect. By bedtime her breathing has become more difficult than ever before. Her mother suggests she should go to bed and try to 'sleep it off'. Petra goes upstairs. She is sweating and thoroughly anxious. She cannot lie down or sleep. She goes to the window thinking to get more air. She finds she can breathe in reasonably well but has the greatest difficulty in breathing out.

Her mother comes upstairs and finds her in great distress and in near-panic. She can hardly speak. The skin around her lips is a blue-purple colour, and her face is pale and clammy.

Petra's father bundles her into a duvet and carries her to the car. He drives her to the casualty department of the local hospital. Fortunately the hospital is receiving.

THE MANAGEMENT IN HOSPITAL

The casualty officer is summoned and she immediately gives Petra an intravenous injection of aminophylline. She is seriously perturbed by Petra's lack of response to this and calls a consultant who agrees to come in. While they are waiting she gives Petra a steroid drug by injection and a drug to widen the air tubes. She also starts oxygen, given through a mask.

In spite of all this, Petra's condition continues to deteriorate and she is soon in grave danger. Repeatedly, she slips into unconsciousness. Her parents are aware of the doctor's distress and are frantic with anxiety. At last the consultant arrives and immediately assesses the situation. Petra is now in a coma. Without wasting a moment, the consultant asks for an endotracheal tube and, using a laryngoscope, passes this down over Petra's tongue and into her larynx. He seals off the airway by inflating the balloon near its tip. He then connects the tube to a mechanical ventilator, which forces oxygen into her lungs, overcoming the tight spasm of her bronchial tubes by sheer pressure. She is connected to a cardiac monitor which shows that her heart is racing and is becoming irregular.

For nearly an hour it is touch and go with Petra. But, in the end, all the bronchial tube muscles suddenly and unexpectedly relax. At first the doctors think that she has had a cardiac arrest, but the monitor shows that her heart action has improved and the pressures in the ventilator indicate that her airway is open. Petra remains in the intensive care unit all night, but by morning she has recovered dramatically and is able to breathe easily without artificial assistance.

THE DOCTOR'S COMMENTS

On the afternoon of the following day, the consultant asks to see Petra's shaken parents, who have been up all night at her bedside. He tells them that, remarkably, Petra appears to have suffered no ill effects from her ordeal. He has had a long talk with her and he does not think there has been any brain damage from oxygen lack. He asks them many questions. Then he informs them that Petra has never been shown how to use an inhaler properly. He points out that the inhaler brought with her to hospital was out of date and was exhausted so that the poor child effectively had no treatment.

He tells them that Petra's asthma has now entered a new and much more serious phase and that he considers it reprehensible that she should constantly be exposed to the dangers of passive smoking in her home. Atopic subjects exposed to other people's cigarette smoke develop rising levels of the particular antibodies (IgE) that bring about asthma attacks. Petra's IgE levels are high and this is almost certainly what has happened to her. If they have no regard for their own health, they should at least have regard for hers.

Speaking more kindly, he explains that the time to stop an asthma attack is at the very beginning. The secret of control is to ensure that attacks are never allowed to develop. To achieve this, two or even three drugs, taken by inhaler, may be needed. They must be clearly aware of when Petra is slipping out of control; this is best ensured by testing her ability to blow out air from her lungs. This is done with a simple device called a peak flow meter. They will be shown how to use it. He emphasizes that they must regard as dangerous any indication that inhaler treatment is having a reduced effect. Such indication must not be ignored. Petra will be taught how to use her inhalers properly and which to use routinely on the first suggestion of breathing difficulty. Treatment must *never* be left until an attack becomes severe. Petra must use the peak flow meter, under supervision, every day.

THE FOLLOW-UP

Although she is only seven, Petra soon becomes expert in the use of her inhalers. She has had a terrible fright and never wants to have such an experience again. Sadly, she agrees to give away her beloved animals to friends. Mr and Mrs Greenwald also make a sacrifice and give up smoking. Petra now knows how to monitor her breathing ability with her peak flow meter and can tell when she must move up to the next level of treatment.

Since her visit to hospital she has never had another severe asthmatic attack.

Does childhood asthma always persist?

Current research shows that 10 per cent of all primary school children in Britain have had a positive diagnosis of asthma. A further 10 to 15 per cent also have symptoms that suggest that they too probably have asthma. These are remarkable figures, but the situation is not so pessimistic as this extraordinarily high incidence might suggest. Most of these children never suffer a really severe attack, and in those relatively mild cases the outlook for a permanent cure of the condition is good.

The *British Medical Journal* of 9 July 1994 carries a report of a major study done to assess which factors in childhood asthma affect the way the disease will progress in later life. This shows that of all the children with asthma at the age of seven, only 25 per cent continued to have asthma as adults. In general, those who continue to suffer are fairly severe asthmatics who, in particular, developed the disease after the age of two. They also tend to be female, to have atopy – especially eczema (see chapter 2) – and to have parents who also suffer from asthma.

In children who do not continue to suffer asthma, the trouble usually settles down in the teens.

Is it really asthma?

Many cases of asthma in children are never recognized for what they are. This is partly because there are a number of conditions that cause similar symptoms, and it is often assumed that it is these, rather than asthma, from which the child is suffering. The diagnosis is especially difficult in very young children whose air tubes are naturally so narrow that they are very easily partly obstructed. A quite mild attack of a cold or bronchitis will readily produce enough mucus in the airways to cause a dramatic wheeze. This is well known to doctors, and although the effect closely resembles the symptoms of asthma, there is a tendency to assume that the trouble is no more than a respiratory tract infection. Doctors are not particularly keen to frighten parents with a firm diagnosis of asthma at such an early age. In addition, they know that most wheezes in very young children do not indicate serious trouble.

Follow-up studies, however, show that of all children under one year of age who develop occasional wheezing, more than 30 per cent have asthma later in childhood. Wheezing that occurs later, when the air tubes have developed and enlarged, must always be regarded as asthma until a convincing alternative is proved. It is surprising how many children have frequent episodes of wheezing without the diagnosis of asthma ever being considered.

Another difficulty is that some cases of genuine asthma start with very little wheezing, but instead feature repeated attacks of coughing. These attacks are liable to occur at bedtime. Such children are usually labelled as suffering from bronchitis and are often treated with antibiotics. Even when wheezing and breathlessness supervene, the diagnosis may not be changed. It is only when asthma is suspected and properly treated that everything settles down. In view of the known statistics of childhood asthma, it is obvious that this diagnosis should be considered far more often than it actually is. Attacks of asthma are *far more common* than attacks of bronchitis in young children, and yet bronchitis is diagnosed more often. Repeated attacks of bronchitis imply that the condition has become established and should be called chronic bronchitis. This is actually very rare in children and is hardly ever diagnosed by paediatric specialists.

If there is a family history of atopy (see chapter 2), the diagnosis of asthma, rather than bronchitis, is even more likely to be correct.

Trigger factors in childhood asthma

Several of the many possible factors that start an attack of asthma are especially common in children. Some of these are not widely known. One of them – atmospheric pollution – is also responsible for a substantial increase in the incidence and severity of asthma, especially in children.

Exercise

In most children with asthma, an attack can be triggered by nothing more than exercise. This is easily tested for. We have seen that a characteristic of asthma is the difficulty in blowing out air rapidly. The term used to describe the maximum rate at which a person can exhale is the *peak expiratory flow rate*. This is simply a measure of the maximum speed at which air can flow out of the lungs, and it is easily measured using a simple peak flow meter (see chapters 6 and 7). Obviously, if the air tubes are narrowed by tightening of the wall muscles, it is going to be harder to achieve the normal rate of maximum outward flow. And a reduction in this maximum rate may exist even if there is no apparent problem with breathing out quietly.

Research has shown that in 80 per cent of asthmatic children, running about for five minutes or so will reduce the measured peak expiratory flow rate by more than 15 per cent. This measured reduction comes on within five to ten minutes of the exertion and has nothing to do with the normal breathlessness that results from the exercise. Children who do not suffer from asthma show no reduction in the peak expiratory flow rate after exercise.

This test is often used to confirm or deny the suspicion of asthma in children.

Change in temperature

Children are not usually very subjective and often fail to note, or comment on, matters that affect them. So it is perhaps not particularly surprising that it does not seem to be widely appreciated that a change in environmental temperature – as in going from a warm classroom to a cold exterior – is a potent trigger of an asthmatic attack. Surprisingly, cold dry air, rather than cold damp, is especially likely to provoke an attack in children. (See also chapter 3, pp. 29–30.)

Emotional upset and anxiety

There are all kinds of emotions, pleasurable and otherwise, and any of these can trigger an asthmatic attack in children. Children are usually quick to respond emotionally to changing circumstances and will often range over the gamut of emotions – from misery to high joyful excitement – in a very short time. Any of these emotions can trigger an asthmatic attack.

Asthma is, of course, a profound cause of emotional upset in itself. This is so important that a whole chapter has been devoted to it (see chapter 9).

Atmospheric pollution

This is a most important trigger factor affecting many children, but especially those in inner-city areas where traffic density is high. (The subject is covered in chapter 3.)

Passive smoking

There is a close correlation between the rise in smoking among young women and the rise in the prevalence of asthma in children. Since infants spend most of their time in the home, they are exposed less than are older children to the kind of atmospheric pollutant described above. But if the parents, especially the mother, smoke cigarettes the children are exposed to a form of local atmospheric pollution that is almost certainly as dangerous to them as that in the streets. Research has shown that infant lung function is adversely affected by maternal smoking even before the child is born. Smoking during the pregnancy has been shown to have this effect. After birth, the effect of cigarette smoke particles in the atmosphere is even worse, and this effect may be apparent as early as the first two weeks of life. All the experts now agree that inhaled cigarette smoke increases the tendency of the air tubes to react to other triggers of asthma.

It is an easy matter to take a small sample of blood from the umbilical cord at the time of birth and to check the levels of IgE present. Remarkably, on the basis of this, it is possible to predict with reasonable accuracy whether or not the child will develop allergic problems later. Maternal smoking during pregnancy is associated with a significant rise in the IgE levels in the cord blood. Parental smoking is associated with an earlier onset of asthma, higher rates of the disease and increased need for treatment. Exposure to tobacco smoke is an environmental hazard from which all children should be protected.

Aeroallergens

Doctors interested in asthma are much concerned with what they call *aeroallergens*. An aeroallergen is any substance to which a person may be allergic which can be carried by the air. They include all the fine particle substances, such as pollens, fungal spores, starch granules and house dust mite droppings, that can be carried by the air and inhaled. They also include any chemical substance, whether in the form of solid particles, liquid droplet or gas, that can be transported by the air (see chapter 3). Out-of-doors, aeroallergens are moved by the wind and particulate allergens may be carried long distances. Indoors, they tend to be airborne only briefly, as when domestic dusting or vacuum cleaning is done or when duvets, pillows or bedcovers are shaken.

Any substance to which an atopic child may be allergic can trigger off an attack of asthma. In the home, the most important of these are the excretory products of house dust mites.

Children and house dust mites

There are several different species of house mite but by far the commonest one in Britain, and in many other countries, is *Dermatophagoides pteronyssinus*. In the USA, the commonest house dust mite seems to be *Dermatophagoides farinae*. If you are a Greek scholar you will at once recognize that this genus of mite lives by eating skin. *Derma-* comes from a Greek root relating to 'skin' and *phago-* comes from the Greek word *phagein*, meaing 'to eat'. These tiny microscopic creatures – they are no more than 0.5 millimetres (0.02 inches) long, are very widely distributed throughout the Western world and live in bedding, mattresses, soft furniture, soft toys, upholstery and carpets. They are very particular as to their diet and live on the scales of human and animal skin that are constantly being shed.

When these mites were first suspected of causing allergy it was assumed that it was their body parts that were allergenic. Later it was shown that the allergen was in the mite droppings, and later still that the real allergen was a protein that coats the droppings. This protein is a digestive enzyme used by the mite to break down the protein of the skin scales so that the mites can use the products. Now that we know the real cause of the trouble we can measure the amounts of this enzyme in house dust samples and thus get a useful idea of the size of the risk in any particular household.

It is easy to discover whether or not a child has become sensitized to dust mite protein. Those who have will have produced IgE antibodies to it and this is readily shown by a skin reaction to a needle prick through a drop of a weak solution of the allergen.

Atopy and the house dust mite protein

Research has shown that, in Britain, the great majority of school children with asthma are already sensitized to the house dust mite protein. A paper in the *New England Journal of Medicine* (23 August 1990) reports a study of 93 British families with children born in 1977 or 1978. In all cases, one parent had asthma or hay fever. The trial started in 1979 and in this year house dust samples were taken. By 1989, 67 of the children were still available for examination, and their homes were visited and further dust samples taken. Of these children, 35 were atopic (see chapter 2) and 32 were not. Seventeen of these children (25 per cent of the total) were found to have active asthma and of these 16 were atopic. All 16 were sensitized to house dust mite protein. All but one of the children with asthma had been exposed at one year of age to substantial levels of dust mite protein. The researchers concluded that, in addition to genetic factors (atopy), exposure to house dust mite allergens in early childhood was an important factor in the subsequent development of asthma.

Because of changes in house furnishings, such as fitted carpets, soft chair coverings and cushions, and because of central heating, house dust mites are much more prevalent in today's homes than they used to be. Mites breed most enthusiastically at temperatures between 18° and 21°C (65° to 70°F), and prefer a relative humidity of at least 50 per cent.

The fact that the main allergen is on the mite droppings is important, because the balls of faeces are relatively heavy and do not float in the air as do smaller and lighter particles such as pollen grains. They do, however, become airborne for half an hour or so if bedding is shaken, or during household cleaning. The use of vacuum cleaners (through which these faecal balls can usually pass) also causes a brief airborne episode. These are the main ways in which this particular dangerous allergen gets into the lungs of children and others.

Remember the soft toys

It has been found that children's soft toys are commonly heavily infested with *D. pteronyssinus*, so it is not particularly surprising that atopic children should develop asthmatic attacks for no obvious reason. Examination of such toys shows that the number of mites on a given area is commonly two and a half times as great as a bed mattress. Here is a useful tip, however. A very effective and safe way of killing mites on soft toys such as teddy bears, so that they are no longer able to produce their protein allergen, is to put the toy in the freezer and leave it for a few hours. Teddy bears come out quite happily and soon warm up because they don't have enough water in them to freeze solid. They soon recover from the experience: but the mites don't.

Studies have also shown that mites are more prevalent if a bedroom is occupied by more than one child and if the bedroom is damp. The house mites' requirement for fluid is illustrated by the fact that they cannot survive in Alpine regions at altitudes above 1,500 metres. At such altitudes, the air is so dry that mites are killed. House dust mite asthma is unknown in these regions.

5
Taking control

This is the most important message of this book. Taking control is what it is all about. People do die of asthma; they are asphyxiated because of blockage of their air tubes. Virtually all these deaths are preventable, but they still occur year after year. The reason for this is simple. Asthma is a treacherous condition. Over the months and years sufferers get accustomed to having recurrent attacks of wheezing. They learn to live with them, and in so doing, soon reach the stage at which familiarity breeds unconcern. When asthma begins to worsen it often does so almost imperceptibly. This is the point at which the danger starts. For worsening asthma can suddenly produce an attack of unprecedented severity.

People who die from asthma either do so out of hospital or get to hospital in such a critical condition that even the application of the most advanced available treatment cannot save them. These disasters happen because no one – neither the sufferer nor parents, nor, occasionally, even the doctor – has really grasped that the asthma is getting worse.

Some facts about death from asthma

Men die from asthma as often as women. About 40 per cent of those who die are below the age of 45. About one third of them did not consider themselves to be particularly severe cases and were free of symptoms for at least three months in the year prior to their death. About 30 per cent did not consider themselves to have chronic asthma, but 40 per cent of them had had previous sudden severe attacks. About 30 per cent of those who die have had a recent severe attack that, in retrospect, is seen to have been badly assessed or badly treated. Some 10 per cent die after stopping, or too rapidly reducing, their dosage of steroids by mouth. About 60 per cent have an atopic tendency (see chapter 2). Only a very small proportion – about 3 per cent – have previously required mechanical assistance with their breathing.

One important and worrying fact is that fatal attacks of asthma may be very brief. In some cases only minutes elapse between the onset of the attack and death. This is unusually brief, however, and the duration of the final attack varies from minutes to days. In 25 per cent of cases, death occurs within an hour of the apparent onset of the attack. A doctor or ambulance is called in less than half of the cases of people who die from asthma. Many of these victims die in private cars on the way to hospital.

These gloomy facts are not meant to depress you but to emphasize the fact that an unusually severe asthmatic attack should be considered to be a medical emergency. It is only too obvious that many asthmatics seriously underestimate the dangers of their disease. Another important fact that a number of studies have brought out is that many deaths could have been prevented if patients understood the value of steroid drugs during the period of gradual deterioration. Doctors who know most about asthma treatment are now convinced that steroids by inhalation and, if necessary, by mouth or injection, are seriously underused when danger threatens. It is tragic that lives should be lost because of an unjustified fear of side-effects. You can read all about the pros and cons of steroid treatment in chapter 7. All in all, in the opinion of the asthma specialists of the British Thoracic Association, 86 per cent of asthma deaths are avoidable and 3 per cent doubtfully avoidable. All these figures have to be regarded as approximations because some of the patients are found dead, and it is not always possible to get adequate details of the previous medical history.

No cause for panic

None of this should be taken as a cause for panic. Of the three million people in Britain with asthma about 2,000 die each year. That is about one person in 1,500 asthmatics – a small proportion of the total. But every death from asthma is an avoidable tragedy and you must ensure that you, or your child, do not add to these distressing statistics. The way to do this is to ensure that you are capable of detecting the danger signs of worsening. This is so basic to the whole business of asthma control that the next chapter is devoted entirely to it.

Research published in the *British Medical Journal* has shown that about 60 per cent of asthma sufferers are not well capable of judging worsening of asthma on the basis of symptoms alone. What is really at issue is the ability to judge narrowing or widening of the air tubes and its effect on the peak flow of air. This research involved 255 asthmatic people between the ages of 17 and 76, from varying environments and social classes. Objective information as to the actual peak flow was obtained using peak flow meters and this was compared with the patients' own subjective judgement of their condition.

One snag is that when an attack seems to be passing off, the person concerned is so relieved that he or she immediately misjudges the residual degree of air flow reduction. Tests show that most asthmatics, when recovering from a severe attack, believe their condition to be normal – as judged by their symptoms – when in fact the air flow is still below 50 per cent of what is normal. Other tests have shown that a great many asthmatics can be given a drug that produces substantial narrowing of the air tubes without their being aware of the fact.

There is an important lesson to be learned from all this. *You cannot safely rely on symptoms alone to assess asthma*. What you must do is actually *measure* peak air flow rates. This is the only way to be sure of what is happening, and this is why the peak flow meter is so important to people with asthma.

Taking control means:

- being aware at all times of the state of the asthma – whether stable or deteriorating;
- using the various medications intelligently so as to ensure, if possible, that the asthma does not get worse;
- responding to any indications of deterioration by stepping up treatment in a prescribed manner;
- reporting urgently to your doctor any suggestion that the asthma might be going out of control.

CASE HISTORY

After studying pharmacology at university Jacquetta became a Member of the Pharmaceutical Society and worked for a time as a community pharmacist. For nine years she has been a hospital pharmacist much valued by her medical colleagues for her helpful advice on drug treatment. Jacquetta is an unusual asthma patient in that she probably knows more about asthma and its management than the average GP. Here is an outline of her case history which illustrates an excellent example of taking control.

PERSONAL DETAILS
Name: Jacquetta Goldberg
Age: 39
Occupation: Hospital pharmacist
Family: Mother and one brother are asthmatic. Father alive and well.

MEDICAL BACKGROUND
Jacquetta showed her atopic tendency at the age of nine months when she developed mild infantile eczema. This troubled her on and off until around puberty but was never severe. Unfortunately, she also developed a marked intermittent wheeze before she was two years old. Initially diagnosed as bronchitis, this was shown by another doctor to be allergic asthma. Jacquetta has the misfortune to be allergic to several allergens and, throughout her childhood, has had many quite severe asthmatic attacks. Unfortunately, the asthma persisted into adult life.

She has established an excellent relationship of mutual respect with the Department of Respiratory Medicine in her hospital and has immediate access to the specialists there. She uses her peak flow meter night and morning, under precisely standardized conditions, and keeps careful documentation of the readings which she records on a monthly graph. She is thus able to check that the variation from morning to night remains small. In the last three weeks she has noticed a slight but definite reduction in her expiratory peak flow rate to about 85 per cent of her normal best. She is watching this closely and is planning to add beclomethasone by inhaler if this drops to 80 per cent.

THE PRESENT COMPLAINT
Jacquetta has the additional misfortune to be sensitive to a number of drugs, including aspirin and several of the non-steroidal anti-inflammatory drugs (NSAIDs). She has to be particularly careful when dispensing these to avoid inhaling loose powder from the bulk storage jars. The care with which she tips out these tablets is proverbial in the dispensary, and her assistants, aware of the problem, are also careful.

One day a new assistant, working alongside her, is dispensing Brufen tablets for a case of rheumatoid arthritis. She has forgotten about Jacquetta's allergy and shakes the open and nearly empty jar vigorously. Within minutes, Jacquetta is wheezing and in a short time she is unable to continue working. She retires to a side room and starts high-dose inhaled beclomethasone via a large-volume spacer device (see chapter 8).

Half an hour later Jacquetta is still wheezing so she adds inhalation of the beta-agonist drug salbutamol (Ventolin) by inhaler. Unfortunately, this too fails to terminate the attack and Jacquetta, with difficulty, telephones a chest consultant and is admitted to the ward.

THE MANAGEMENT IN HOSPITAL

No time is wasted. Jacquetta is given an intravenous injection of prednisolone and another of aminophylline. She is also given oxygen by mask and arrangements are made for an anaesthetist to be on hand to pass a tracheal tube, should this prove necessary. Fortunately, the injections are sufficient and the acute stage passes quickly. Jacquetta is prescribed steroids by mouth to be taken for a period of a few weeks and then tapered off. She does not have to be told that it is dangerous suddenly to stop steroids, but she is told all the same.

Jacquetta is back at work the next day.

6
How to detect the danger signs

CASE HISTORY

Martin had been asthmatic since he was four. Both he and his mother are knowledgeable on the subject and are aware of the danger signs. Once a week Martin checks his peak flow reading. One day he finds that this is reduced to about 80 per cent of the normal figure and wisely suggests that he should see his doctor.

PERSONAL DETAILS

Name: Martin Kaplan
Age: 17
Occupation: Student
Family: Both parents alive and well. Two sisters. Both suffer from eczema and hay fever.

MEDICAL BACKGROUND

Martin's asthma is allergic. His atopic tendency is inherited. The same cause led to his suffering from eczema as a child, but that has now cleared up. His attacks vary greatly in severity, ranging from mild breathlessness, sometimes brought on by exercise, and a feeling of tightness in the chest, to severe attacks of wheezing, dry cough, sweating, rapid heart beat, and distress and anxiety. Martin uses two kinds of inhaler – one containing a bronchodilator drug and, when necessary, another containing a corticosteroid.

THE CONSULTATION WITH THE FAMILY DOCTOR

Martin tells the doctor that he has been using both inhalers, but that they seem to be losing their effect. The doctor commends Martin for his promptness in reporting the drop in the peak flow reading, reminding him, unnecessarily, that the apparent loss of effectiveness of routine treatment is a danger sign.

Examination shows that Martin is breathing a little more quickly than normal and that, although he can breathe in easily, he is having some difficulty in breathing out. As a result, his chest remains more fully expanded than normal. A meter test confirms that Martin's peak flow rate is markedly reduced. During the consultation Martin develops a severe attack. He is unable to lie down and soon is hardly able to speak. The difficulty in getting enough oxygen into his blood results in cyanosis – a bluish-purple discoloration of his face, particularly his lips.

THE DIAGNOSIS AND COMMENTS

Martin's asthma control has deteriorated and he is liable to pass into a state in which treatment is much more difficult. He urgently needs more effective medication to control the progressive tendency to spasm of the muscles in his bronchial tubes. The doctor decides that he had better be admitted to hospital for intensive treatment. While waiting for the ambulance, the doctor gives him an intravenous injection of aminophylline.

THE TREATMENT

In hospital this drug is repeated and he is given oxygen by mask. There is little response so he is given adrenaline, also by intravenous injection. Martin's breathing becomes a little easier, but the attack is not controlled until he is given a large dose of corticosteroids by injection. This is followed by a tapering schedule of steroids and he is soon fully recovered. The doctors had contemplated giving him forced oxygen under pressure, but this was not required.

THE FOLLOW-UP

Martin is now even more aware than before of the importance of monitoring the state of his bronchial tubes. He remains optimistic as he knows that half of affected young people grow out of asthma completely by the age of 21 and that in a proportion of the remainder, attacks become decreasingly severe as they grow older. He also knows that, with good drug treatment, even people who suffer repeated attacks as adults can expect to live an almost normal life. He is heartened by the knowledge that several world-class athletes suffer from asthma.

The peak expiratory flow meter

No one is now in any doubt as to the very real advantages of peak flow monitoring. Chest physicians have recognized for many years the predictive value of these simple devices in providing asthmatics with warning of deterioration. There is now a very strong case for the view that everyone using an inhaler for asthma should also be using a peak flow meter.

Background

Tests of lung function by measuring forced expiration have been in use for a long time by experts in hospital. These tests originally measured the *volume* of the expired air in a given time. To do this they required cumbersome apparatus called recording spirometers in which large hollow pistons, with counter-balancing weights to reduce their resistance and inertia, were caused to move in cylinders, blown along by the volume of the forced expiration. This equipment was expensive, cumbersome and delicate, but the value of these tests was considerable. Research showed that the volume of air breathed out in the first second of a forced expiration, after taking the fullest possible breath, was a reliable indication of the respiratory performance for a much longer period – up to 15 seconds. This was so both in people with normal lungs and in those with asthma.

This volume, known as the peak expiratory volume (PEV_1), is normally more than 70 per cent of the full capacity of the lungs (the *vital capacity*). Vital capacity is defined as the maximum volume of air that can be breathed out after taking a full inspiration. In asthma, the forced expiratory volume, in the first second, is markedly reduced – commonly to only half the normal value and often to a much lower figure.

Peak expiratory flow

There is no way to measure peak expiratory *volume* directly without taking up a lot of space. Many people have a vital capacity of four litres, so the equipment must be at least this voluminous. Fortunately, in asthma, there is a close relationship between the value of the peak expiratory volume in the first second (the PEV_1) and the maximum air flow *rate* at the beginning of a forced expiration. This maximum rate is called the *peak expiratory flow rate* (PEFR). You can measure peak flow rate with a very simple, portable and cheap device called a peak flow meter. So one of the most generally practicable tests of the ease or difficulty with which air can pass along the air tubes of the lung is now the measurement of the peak expiratory flow rate.

It is most important that peak flow meters should be used properly (see below). The readings are a good indication of the severity of the airway obstruction. The measurement is especially useful for detecting worsening of asthma and assessing the response to treatment.

Why use peak flow meters?

As we have seen in the last chapter, subjective assessments of breathlessness are a very unreliable guide to the state of the calibre of the air tubes and to the volume of the airflow. The degree of wheezing can be very misleading in this respect. It may be pronounced in moderate cases and almost absent in very severe cases. What we really want to know is the ease with which air can pass in and out of the lungs. The peak flow meter can give us a reliable, objective assessment of this.

This is very important because deteriorating performance is dangerous and may be followed by a severe, and perhaps potentially fatal, attack. This cannot be too often emphasized. Nearly all the lives claimed by asthma could be saved if effective treatment could be given at an early stage to prevent sudden and severe worsening. A reducing air-flow performance is a clear sign that changes in treatment are needed to improve control. Regular monitoring can, for instance, demonstrate increasing differences between morning and evening peak expiratory flow rates – a hint that control is inadequate. Properly informed people with asthma, provided with this kind of objective indication of their air-flow status, can, by themselves, make appropriate changes in their treatment – such as adding or increasing steroids (see chapter 7) – or can seek medical help urgently.

Like people with diabetes, people with asthma should know at all times what is going on in their bodies and should be clearly aware of the principles of treatment. Peak flow rate figures in asthmatics can be considered as analogous to blood sugar readings in diabetics. The main difference, however, is that oxygen lack is far more immediately dangerous than a rise in blood sugar. Many asthmatics are too young to be able to assess their own condition. In these cases, someone else – usually a parent – must do it for them.

Peak flow readings are also important in monitoring the effect of a *reduction* in treatment when it is thought that a patient is possibly being overtreated. Reduction in steroid dosage, for instance, can only safely be achieved if the effect of the change on peak air flow is assessed at the time.

What do patients think?

It has been suggested that some patients might become neurotic about their peak flow readings. This may be so, but this is hardly an argument against the procedure. The great majority are only too pleased to have the constant reassurance, and the sense of personal involvement and control, that the method provides. In one research trial, patients regularly using inhalers were told about the usefulness and cost of peak flow meters and were asked whether they would be interested in buying one. Of the 163 patients who replied to the questionnaire, 53 (33 per cent) said they already had a meter and 70 (43 per cent) said they would be interested in buying one. Of those who were not interested, the main reasons given were that their asthma was not severe enough (25 per cent), or was well controlled (22 per cent), or that they could not afford the meter (22 per cent).

How to use a peak flow meter

The best results from peak flow meters are obtained from children over the age of six years and from adults. In measuring PEFR you, or the child, should stand upright, take a full breath and make as rapid and forceful an expiration as possible. The meter should be held horizontally. Be sure that the lips make a proper seal around the mouthpiece of the meter. Any leakage of air around the mouthpiece or any air that passed out through the nose will, of course, give a falsely low reading. Don't practise too often before taking the definitive readings. Repeated deep breathing (hyperventilation) before the test can produce an artificially low result. Some children become adept at producing a fraudulently high value by 'air spitting', or by ballooning out their cheeks and suddenly releasing the air through the meter. These trick methods can be dangerously misleading and should not be allowed. Three measurements should be performed each time and the best result accepted. Ignore any results that seem improbably low – accept only constant and consistent results.

It is necessary to know what the normal reading should be for any individual, so that abnormal readings can be detected. The best way to do this is to take lots of readings at different times when the person concerned is perfectly well and to accept as normal the figures that are consistently highest. In children, peak expiratory flow rate (PEFR) increases uniformly with height. A rough idea of the normal for any given child can be got from the following table:

Height (in cm.)	*PEFR* (in litres per minute)
100	100
110	150
120	200
130	250
140	300
150	350
160	400
170	450

These figures are approximate only. The child's best performance in health is a more useful guide.

Peak flow readings should be recorded. You can make up your own charts or, in Britain, you can use the charts provided by the Department of Health (reference number FP1010). Many people prefer the more elegant record cards or diaries provided by drug companies, but you must remember that peak flow meter monitoring is a long-term matter and you are going to need plenty of cards. There is much to be said for the 'official' record card and you may find it easier to maintain a reliable supply if you use FP1010s.

The peak flow meter plan

Point 1 You have to know what your normal, or desirable, peak flow really is. You do this by keeping careful records and seeing what you, or your child, can do when perfectly well and free from symptoms. This figure is not necessarily the best possible result, but it should be close to it. It is the figure you can consistently maintain when well.

Point 2 You should continue with your normal routine treatment so long as the peak flow reading is somewhere between 80 per cent and 100 per cent of this figure.

Point 3 If the peak flow reading falls below 80 per cent of normal, see your doctor without delay because *you need extra treatment*. This may involve additional β_2 agonist doses (see chapter 7) to widen your air tubes, or extra steroid inhalation. It may even require that you start a course of steroid tablets. Your doctor will advise on this. Some people taking inhaled steroids routinely double the dose if the peak flow reading falls below 80 per cent of normal. Many do this routinely at the first sign of a cold.

Point 4 If the peak flow falls below 50 per cent *you are in the medical alert zone and are in danger*. Step up your self-treatment and *get to your doctor immediately*. Tell your doctor that your peak flow reading is less than 50 per cent of normal.

7
How to treat asthma

Although it is true that you can never know too much about asthma and about its management, you should not infer from this that asthma control is entirely a do-it-yourself matter. Every person with asthma needs professional medical attention. It is no part of the purpose of this book to dictate a particular scheme of treatment for you. That is the job of your doctor.

There are, however, established principles in asthma treatment that are accepted by almost all doctors and these you should understand. The first thing you need to know about are the different classes of drugs used: how they differ in their action; their advantages and disadvantages; their possible side-effects; and when they are used. You will be relieved to learn that there are only a few relevant drug groups and that the members of each group are more or less interchangeable.

Beta$_2$ (β_2) adrenoreceptor agonists

Don't let this complicated heading put you off; it is not nearly so difficult as it sounds. First the word *agonist*. You know what an antagonist is – somebody or something that is against someone or something else. An agonist is something that acts in the same way as something else. *Adrenoreceptor* simply means a place or site at which adrenaline acts. Adrenaline is, of course, the natural body hormone that is poured into the bloodstream in times of emergency. It is the hormone of fright, fight and flight. One of the things needed when fighting or fleeing is wide open air tubes in the lungs. And this is one of the useful effects of adrenaline. In fact, adrenaline works very well in asthma, but it is not routinely used because it has so many other effects, some of them rather unpleasant. An adreno-receptor agonist is a drug that has much the same effect as adrenaline in relaxing the muscles in the walls of the air tubes and so widening them.

Fortunately, because of the many effects of adrenaline, there are half a dozen different kinds of adrenoreceptors. Some act on the heart and the arteries; some even cause smooth muscle to *tighten*.

There are $alpha_1$ and $alpha_2$ receptors and $beta_1$ and $beta_2$ receptors.

Of these, the receptors that people with asthma are interested in are the $beta_2$ (β_2) receptors. This is because the β_2 receptors are on the smooth muscles that run around the walls of the air tubes in the lungs. Anything that stimulates these receptors causes the muscles to relax and the tubes to widen. Pharmacists have been very busy producing drugs that act like adrenaline but only affect the β_2 receptors. These are the $beta_2$ adrenergic agonists – drugs that act like adrenaline. The most commonly used β_2 agonists are salbutamol (Ventolin, Salamol, Salbulin), terbutaline (Bricanyl), rimiterol (Pulmadil) and fenoterol (Duovent).

Drugs that attach to the beta receptors and stay there but without stimulating them into action are called 'beta-blockers'. These are very useful in other branches of medicine as they can slow down an overactive heart and reduce high blood pressure. Beta-blockers are beta receptor *antagonists* and when they act on the β_2 receptors they have exactly the *opposite* effect that is wanted by anyone suffering from asthma. So drugs like propranolol (Inderal) or oxprenolol (Trasicor), indeed any of the beta-blocker drugs, are very dangerous for people with asthma (see chapter 11).

The 'rebound' phenomenon

One of the snags with the β_2 agonist drugs is that, although they are very effective immediately, and have a useful action for up to about six hours, something very undesirable may happen thereafter. In people using them regularly, the period following the wearing off of the air tube widening effect often features an *increased* tendency for a further attack to be triggered off. This increased sensitivity (*reactivity*) is called a 'rebound' effect, and it can, of course be dangerous. All too easily, it can start a kind of vicious spiral in which the β_2 agonist drug is overused. This raises the important question of the safety of these drugs.

Are β_2 agonists safe?

There is something else you should know about β_2 agonists. In the 1960s, after the introduction of a high-dose isoprenaline preparation, available over the counter, a virtual epidemic of asthma deaths occurred in Britain. There was, naturally, a good deal of adverse publicity and this preparation was withdrawn. Isoprenaline is a non-selective beta receptor agonist. That means that it stimulates not only the β_2 receptors but also the β_1 receptors. Because of this it greatly speeds up the heart causing palpitations, heart irregularity and, in some people, angina pectoris.

Another epidemic occurred in New Zealand after the introduction of a high-dose preparation of the drug fenoterol. This drug is more selective for the β_2 receptors than for the β_1 receptors, but it still has some stimulant effect on the latter. Taken in high dosage it can have the same effects as those described from isoprenaline. Research done at the time indicated that more of the people who died from asthma were taking fenoterol than other β_2 agonists. Again, the number of deaths dropped after the high-dose preparation was withdrawn.

No one has been able to explain these two epidemics of asthma deaths, but they do seem to have been connected with the use of the high-dose β_2 agonists. Presumably the β_1 receptor effects have much to do with it, and it is possible also that the rebound phenomenon (see above) may also be involved. But the people who died, did so from *asthma* not from heart trouble. There is some evidence that as a person acquires tolerance to a ß adrenergic agonist drug the asthma may deteriorate. It has to be said, however, that epidemics of asthma deaths have occurred independently of the use of these drugs. It is also rather strange that epidemic deaths did not occur in countries other than Britain and New Zealand where the same drugs were being taken. Other trials have failed to show that long-term use of β_2 agonists causes a reduction in lung function.

There is one ingenious possible explanation: people whose asthma is severe and worsening are more likely to be using high doses of β_2 agonists as these are highly effective in relieving attacks. This group of people are also the most likely to die from asthma. Looked at in this way, it is wrong to assume that the β_2 agonist drugs are necessarily the cause of the increased deaths.

Whatever the truth of the matter, the moral is clear. Don't be too casual about this particular class of drugs. Inhaled β_2 agonists are valuable drugs used by millions of asthma sufferers. But you should appreciate that when you use them you are treating the symptoms of asthma, not the underlying cause of the disease. β_2 agonists have no effect on the inflammation which is such an important part of the basic problem, nor do they in any way influence the immune system disorder. If your asthma is getting worse, this is very definitely *not* a reason to increase your use of your β_2 agonist inhaler. What you need is an increased use of inhaled steroids or perhaps another kind of air tube widening drug such as ipratropium (Atrovent) or theophylline (Labophylline, Lasma, Nuelin, Theo-Dur).

The basic difference between β_2 receptor agonists and other asthma drugs

β_2 receptor agonists are normally used as the first-line treatment of an asthmatic attack. This means that they are used at irregular intervals and often on an 'as required' basis. This fact may lead you to suppose that the other drugs used in asthma management may also be used intermittently. This would be a serious mistake. In this sense, there is a basic difference between the beta stimulators and steroids, cromoglycate and ipratropium bromide (see below). These drugs must be taken properly, usually four times a day, over an extended period. They should never be used 'as required'.

All about steroids

The group of steroid drugs, known medically as the corticosteroids, were developed from the natural body hormone cortisol, produced by the outer layer (cortex) or the adrenal gland. In fact, the first steroid drug, cortisone, *was* natural hormone. A steroid is a member of the large chemical group of sterols, related to fats, which includes cholesterol, bile acids, sex hormones, and the adrenal cortex hormones. Corticosteroid drugs are all chemically similar to the natural steroid hormones.

These drugs have many uses in medicine and have saved many lives. When used for asthma they can be taken by inhalation or by mouth, or given by injection. They are highly effective against inflammation and in suppressing other functions of the immune system that can be dangerous or damaging. But, as is usually the case, powerful drugs nearly always have major side-effects, and the corticosteroids, given in large dosage, are no exception. But you must view this with a sense of proportion and not allow yourself to be frightened off steroids by tales of serious side-effects. Remember that steroids used in an inhaler are very unlikely to have any significant general side-effects, as the dose is very small and, properly used, the drug goes only where it is needed.

Steroids are invaluable in asthma. Among their many useful effects are that they:

- cut the inflammation in the air tubes;

- reduce mucus secretion;
- reduce the number of mast cells in the air tube lining;
- improve the action of β_2 agonists (see above);
- reduce the amount of IgE produced in the body (see chapter 2);
- reduce the amount of histamine and other irritants produced;
- interfere with T cell interleukin production (see below).

In the past, doctors have tended to avoid prescribing steroids for asthma, but it is now recognized that, so far as asthma is concerned, under-prescribing of steroids is more dangerous than over-prescribing. Today, the advice of the experts – who are better informed than most of the possible dangers of steroids – is strongly in favour of using inhaled steroids, when needed, rather than trying to avoid them.

Between 3 and 5 per cent of people with asthma, however, need steroids in doses larger than can be obtained from inhalers. Such dosage is not ordered lightly and it is given because it is necessary to control otherwise severe symptoms. The risks of *not* taking sufficiently large doses are far greater than the risks of the possible side-effects. Whether or not you are in this category, you should be aware of what can happen if steroids are taken in high doses for long periods. Such doses will inevitably cause some side-effects. These vary with the dose and how the drug is given. But if enough steroid gets into the body there is a chance that one or more of the following effects may occur:

- suppression of the body's production of natural steroids;
- reactivation of latent infections such as tuberculosis;
- an increased susceptibility to new infections, such as thrush;
- the breakdown of partly-healed stomach or duodenal ulcers;
- osteoporosis;
- diabetes;
- high blood pressure;
- excessive hairiness (hirsutism);
- glaucoma;
- cataract.

These complications are comparatively uncommon and affect people taking steroids by mouth for long periods in doses greater than is usual in the control of asthma. The steroid drugs most commonly given in this way are prednisolone (Prednesol) and methylprednisolone (Medrone).

Suppression of the body's own steroid production

This effect of large-dose steroid treatment will do no harm so long as the amount of steroid being taken is at least as much as the body normally produces, but there is a snag. When steroids are taken as drugs, the body's monitoring system turns off the natural production from the adrenal glands. So if the drug is suddenly stopped there may be little or no steroid in the blood. The effects of this can be very dangerous.

Furthermore, if the body's steroid production is suppressed in this way and an emergency occurs which would normally result in a very large outpouring of steroid from the adrenals, the person concerned might be in very serious danger because of the lack of this sudden large dose. The only thing that might save his or her life would be a large injection or steroid. For this reason, all patients on long-term steroid treatment must carry a card indicating, in detail, the treatment they are having. In the event of a severe accident or other major stress, a doctor would give such an injection.

On average, suppression of natural steroid production can be expected to occur in people taking more than about 7.5 mg of prednisolone per day. Prednisolone is the commonest oral drug used in asthma.

There is one way in which the risk of suppression of natural hormone production can be minimized, and this is widely advised, especially in the USA. The idea is to find out the minimum effective daily dose and then to give 2.5 times this dose before 8 a.m. *on alternate days*. This method is said to reduce substantially the tendency to suppression of adrenal cortisone production. Unfortunately, alternate day therapy may result in inadequate control on the days the drug is not taken. There is no reason, however, why steroids by inhalation should not be taken along with steroids by mouth.

The risks of side-effects of steroids vary considerably from person to person and may be minimal. Doctors, however, will always balance the risks against the disadvantages of not using high-dose, long-term steroids. The decision to give long-term steroids to young children must be balanced against the fact that these drugs cause stunting of growth. There is evidence that doses of inhaled steroid, such as beclomethasone, in excess of 600 to 800 μg per day can cause growth retardation in children. It must be remembered, however, that the same effect may be caused by serious childhood illnesses, for which steroids may be needed. A considerable proportion of the dose of any inhaled medication is always retained in the mouth and throat, so in the case of people having high doses of inhaled steroids it is worth considering washing out the mouth and gargling to eliminate excess steroid after each use of a steroid inhaler and minimize the amount absorbed into the bloodstream. The use of a large volume spacer (see chapter 9) can also reduce the amount deposited in the mouth and throat.

The commonest side-effects of inhaled steroids are thrush infection (*candidiasis*) of the mouth and throat, cough and hoarseness. Established candidiasis can be treated with antifungal gargles or lozenges, or an imidazole preparation by mouth.

Xanthine derivative drugs

The xanthines are the group of drugs that include *caffeine* (coffee, tea, Coca-Cola), *theophylline* and *theobromine* (cocoa, chocolate), as well as a range of substances of similar chemical composition. Caffeine, in the form of strong coffee, has been used to treat asthma for well over a century, but its effect is rather slight. Theobromine has even less effect than caffeine. Theophylline, however, has a strong effect in widening the air passages.

Theophylline is not at all soluble and as a result is poorly absorbed when taken by mouth. But if it is compounded with other substances it can be made soluble. Theophylline ethylene diamine is one such compound. Because it is an amine compound it is usually called aminophylline. This drug, and other soluble theophylline compounds, such as diprophylline, choline theophyllinate (Choledyl) and proxyphilline, are widely used in the treatment of asthma attacks. Once these substances get into the body they are converted to theophylline.

The main action of theophylline is to relax muscle, especially the smooth muscle in the walls of the bronchi. How it does this is still unknown, but the effect is greatest when the muscles are tight. Theophylline also improves the efficiency of the diaphragm – the large domed sheet of muscle between the chest and the abdomen that, with the rib movements, increases the volume of the chest and allows us to inhale air. These respiratory muscles tend to become fatigued during an asthma attack and theophylline reduces this fatigue.

Theophylline, like caffeine, is also an effective stimulator of the central nervous system. This can, unfortunately, limit the dose that is used to treat asthma. Too much can even cause convulsions. The drug is not recommended for people who are prone to panic disorders. The effect on the brain has been used to rouse dying people to a brief, once-only, spell of consciousness and coherence, Other side-effects include:

- nausea;
- vomiting;
- loss of appetite;
- abdominal discomfort;
- hyperactivity;
- personality changes;
- fast pulse;
- heart irregularity.

The dosage of theophylline is fairly critical and must be carefully assessed. Too little, and the effect is very small; too much and undesirable side-effects occur. The dose that causes these side-effects is less than three times the minimal effective dose, so there is little room for manoeuvre. Theophylline is most commonly taken by mouth in tablet form, often formulated as a sustained-release preparation. In severe cases it is given by intravenous injection. The average daily dose is 12 mg per kilo body weight in adults, 16 mg per kilo in children 9 to 16 years old, and 20 mg per kilo in children aged 1 to 9. In infants the dose is calculated on the basis of exact body weight and on the age in months.

The effectiveness of theophylline depends on the levels of the drug achieved in the bloodstream. This varies with a number of other factors and any of these that might be relevant should be noted. Theophylline blood levels are reduced by:

- cigarette smoking;
- a high protein, low carbohydrate diet;
- age under 16;
- eating charcoal-grilled meat;
- various other drugs, including those used to control epilepsy.

It should hardly be necessary to repeat that no asthmatic subject should ever consider cigarette smoking.

Some factors *increase* blood levels of theophylline. These include:

- obesity;
- age over 50 years;
- virus infections;
- influenza A virus vaccination;
- liver disease;
- heart failure;
- oral contraceptives;
- certain drugs, such as cimetidine (Tagamet), erythromycin antibiotics (Erythrocin), ciprofloxacin antibiotics (Ciproxin), allopurinol (Zyloric, Hamarin).

Some of these factors might raise the blood levels above the toxic threshold and precipitate side-effects. People to whom these factors apply should be wary of large doses.

Anticholinergic drugs

Before explaining how these drugs work, it is necessary to say something about a part of the nervous system that is not well understood outside medical circles. This is the part called the *autonomic nervous system*. In spite of the name this is not a separate nervous system but simply a collection of nerves concerned with the automatic and non-voluntary control of many body functions. These nerves lie in clusters, called *ganglia*, situated all the way up and down either side of spine. These ganglia receive connections directly from the adjacent parts of the spinal cord. Some of the autonomic nerves come out directly from the brainstem – the part between the main brain and the spinal cord.

We would be in real trouble without the constant action of the autonomic nervous system. The system has two generally opposing and balancing parts – the sympathetic, concerned with emergency situations (fright, fight and flight), and the parasympathetic, concerned with calm situations. As you will probably have realized, adrenaline is the sympathetic hormone. (If this doesn't make much sense it would be a good idea to go back and read the section on β_2 adrenoreceptor agonists earlier in this chapter). The equivalent hormone in the parasympathetic division of the autonomic is called *acetylcholine*. This hormone is just as powerful as adrenaline but, of course, it works in the opposite direction. To put it crudely, adrenaline is an 'upper'; acetylcholine is a 'downer'.

Acetylcholine has many effects, all of them concerned with the kinds of body activities appropriate to safe, quiet situations. These effects include:

- narrowing (constriction) of the pupils;
- contraction of the bladder-wall;
- relaxation of controlling muscle rings (sphincters);
- the production of saliva, tears, sweat and lung secretions;
- slowing of the heart;
- increasing of the activity of the bowels;
- narrowing of the air tubes.

These acetylcholine effects are called *cholinergic* and it is the last of them that concerns us most in relation to asthma. You may be wondering why we are interested in a system that does the very opposite of what we require. The reason is that if we can find drugs that block the action of the parasympathetic system we should be able to *prevent* the very thing we want to avoid. Drugs that block the receptors for acetylcholine are called *anticholinergic* drugs.

One of these, the very powerful drug *atropine* (belladonna), has been known for a long time as it is found in the deadly nightshade *Atropa belladonna*. It was so called because for centuries it has been known that the juice from the berries will greatly widen (dilate) the pupils of the eyes thereby enhancing female attractiveness. 'Bella donna' is Italian for 'beautiful woman'. Incidentally, atropa comes from the Greek *atropos*, meaning 'unchangeable' – a reference to the tendency for the drug, in excess, to cause death.

Powerful anticholinergic drugs such as atropine have, of course, a wide range of effects which, after consulting the above list of parasympathetic actions, you can work out for yourself. They cause a dry mouth, dry eyes, a dry, hot skin, widely dilated pupils, a rapid hearbeat, relief of bowel colic, difficulty in emptying the bladder and widening of the air passages of the lungs. Atropine was, in fact, used to treat asthma until about the beginning of this century but, as you might imagine, the side-effects made it rather unpopular for this purpose. Another reason why it became unpopular with doctors was that it dried up the lung secretions so that there was a danger that the smaller air tubes might become blocked by mucus plugs. Atropine also interferes with the beating action of the cilia on the tube lining cells (see chapter 1) and there was concern that this would encourage infection.

So, although atropine was largely abandoned as a treatment for asthma, it, and its derivatives, remain valuable for other medical purposes. Anticholinergics are widely used to:

- dry up secretions prior to an operation;
- treat an unduly slow heart rate;
- relieve the symptoms of the irritable bowel syndrome;
- treat some types of urinary incontinence;
- treat Parkinson's disease;
- relieve motion sickness.

Although you are unlikely to encounter the side-effects of these drugs, it would be as well if you were aware of the effects of anticholinergic overdose. This will also help you to remember the actions. In addition to the effects mentioned, overdosage can also cause:

- difficulty in swallowing;
- retention of urine;
- blurred vision;
- anxiety;
- delirium;
- hallucinations;
- confusion and convulsions.

Note how many of these are effects on the brain itself.

Apart from atropine, other anticholinergic drugs are hyoscine (Buscopan), scopolamine (the same as hyoscine), homatropine, banthine, propantheline (Pro-Banthine) and dibutoline. None of these is really suitable for the treatment of asthma because, in the doses needed to have a useful effect on the air tubes, the side-effects would be too severe to be acceptable. Fortunately, this is not the end of the story.

Pharmacologists are always looking for ways of adjusting drugs chemically so that certain actions are enhanced and others suppressed. The value of the relaxing effect of atropine on the smooth muscle of the air tube walls was obviously worth following up. In the mid-1970s one particular change to the atropine molecule was found which had exactly the desired effect. The drug produced in this way is called *ipratropium*, and it is even more powerful than atropine at widening the air tubes. At the same time, it has a much less powerful effect on the brain and, rather surprisingly, very little adverse effect on the cilia of the bronchial tubes. This last feature was a real bonus. Ipratropium can be used without risking the accumulation of secretions in the tubes.

When ipratropium is taken by inhalation, its action is confined almost wholly to the air passages and mouth. Even in dosage many times greater than that required to widen the air passages, the drug produces little or no change in the rate of the heart, the blood pressure or the size of the pupil. The effects on the brain are negligible because less than 1 per cent of the inhaled dose of the drug is absorbed into the circulation.

The performance of ipratropium is impressive. Various things, such as cigarette smoke, ozone, sulphur dioxide, methacholine or other irritants, cause the air tubes of normal people to narrow. Early tests performed on people who were not asthmatic showed that if ipratropium is taken the effects of these irritants were virtually abolished and no narrowing occurred. This was exciting and promised great things for the drug. When ipratropium was tried in people with asthma, the effect, in preventing narrowing of the airways from these same irritant substances, was almost equally dramatic. But the effects on asthma cases generally was less impressive. Research showed that, unfortunately, ipratropium was not particularly effective in preventing narrowing as a result of histamine and other mast cell granule products (see chapter 2). It does, however, have some useful effect on these also.

The effect of the drug in preventing air tube narrowing in response to exercise or breathing cold air varies considerably from person to person and from time to time. This is because of the varying degrees to which the parasympathetic is involved in these stimuli to air tube narrowing. Many asthmatic people find the drug valuable.

Clinical trials have shown that if a β_2 adrenergic agonist (see above) is followed by ipratropium, the two seem to enhance each other. Widening of the air tubes for up to six hours can be obtained in this way. As a result of this observation, inhalers containing a combination of ipratropium with a β_2 agonist such as fenoterol have been produced and are widely used. The British trade name for this preparation is Duovent. Ipratropium has also been produced in a formulation that includes a xanthine drug. The combination of ipratropium and salbutamol is sold under the trade name Combivent.

Another drug chemically very similar to ipratropium and with closely similar effects is oxitropium (Oxivent). The '-vent' ending in all these trade names refers, of course, to the increased 'ventilation' of the lungs produced by the drugs.

Cromoglycate drugs

Sodium cromoglycate (cromolyn) has an interesting history. In 1965 scientists were working on a drug called *khellin* which had been used by the ancient Egyptians as a treatment for colic. Khellin is obtained from the plant *Ammi visnaga*. Chemically, the drug is a benzopyrone or cromone.

Bowel colic is due to tight contraction of the smooth muscle in the walls of the intestine – the same kind of muscle as that in the walls of the air tubes of the lungs. It was hoped that khellin, or a derivative substance, might prove useful as a relaxant of smooth muscle in the walls of the bronchial tubes. Any such effect would widen and open up the airways and thus be effective in asthma. In the course of their work, the scientists synthesized the compound sodium cromoglycate. When this was tried on asthmatics, it proved quite useless as a means of widening the air tubes. Even so, to everyone's surprise, most people with asthma who were given the drug showed a remarkable improvement.

This extraordinary fact was finally explained by the discovery that cromoglycate had another and quite different effect. As explained in chapter 2, allergic asthma results from the release by mast cells of histamine and other highly irritating substances. These act on the smooth muscle in the air tube walls causing it to tighten. In some remarkable way that is still not fully understood, cromolyn acts as if it makes the walls of mast cells stronger so that the granules that contain the irritating substances are not released. The official phrase for this is 'stabilization of the mast cell membrane', but this does not really explain anything. The true action is complicated and involves a change in the effect that the antigen and the IgE have on the cell membrane (see chapter 2).

For practical purposes, you can think of the action of cromoglycate as simply preventing the release of the granule contents. This property is, of course, very valuable for asthmatics. Although cromoglycate does not widen narrowed air tubes, it certainly helps, in this roundabout way, to prevent them from being narrowed. There is another important point. Clinical experience shows that after cromoglycate is used regularly for two or three months there is a definite reduction in the tendency for allergens or exercise to trigger an asthmatic attack.

A good feature of the drug is that it is very poorly absorbed when taken by mouth. Only about 1 per cent actually enters the bloodstream and the small amount absorbed is quickly excreted unchanged in the urine and in the bile. So cromoglycate acts by coming directly into contact with the mast cells in the air tubes. In practice, it is taken by inhalation, either in an aerosol solution or as a powder driven by a turbo inhaler (see chapter 8). For the drug to work properly, therefore, it has to get to the site of its action. This means that the inhaler must be used properly and that the air tubes must be reasonably open before the cromoglycate is taken. So, to achieve adequate dosage, it may be necessary to use a β_2 agonist drug before using the cromoglycate. In some preparations cromoglycate is combined with a β_2 agonist. It is also a good idea, after an effective inhalation of the drug, to hold the breath for a time so as to keep the drug in place for that time rather than simply to blow it out again. Remember that cromoglycate is not an air tube widener and that it is only really effective in cases in which the asthma is allergic in nature.

These facts highlight the importance of understanding as much as possible of the underlying processes of asthma (the *pathology*) and of how these are countered in its treatment. Only in this way can you really take control in an intelligent and reliable manner.

Cromoglycate is sold various trade names (see below). A closely related drug called *nedocromil* has substantially the same properties and is marketed in Britain under the trade name Tilade.

The advancing edge of research

There is still a good deal of doubt as to the mechanisms that cause asthma in the smaller proportion of asthmatic people who are not atopic (see chapter 2). Like those with allergic asthma, these people suffer inflammation of the air tube linings. Mast cells are not a primary feature of this type of asthma and the function of mast cells seems to be taken over by other similar cells called *eosinophils* (see chapter 2). Like mast cells, eosinophils can degranulate and release highly irritating substances. A great deal of attention has, naturally, been given to the eosinophils, and a major advance occurred when the development of fine fibre-optic bronchoscopes made it possible to obtain samples of eosinophils from living patients.

When studying non-allergic asthmatic patients in this way, the scientists found that, along with the eosinophils, there were large numbers of helper T lymphocytes (helper T cells). This was a new departure in asthma research. Helper T cells – the same group of T cells that are attacked by HIV to cause AIDS – had not previously been thought to be involved in asthma. These T cells were found to produce a chemical substance called interleukin-5 that activated the eosinophils and encouraged them to degranulate and release their inflammation-causing substances. Studies on people with allergic asthma showed that a slightly different group of helper T cells were importantly involved in prompting B cells to produce IgE (see chapter 2). They did so by secreting a substance called interleukin-4.

Up to this point, everything you have read has been orthodox science and has been accepted by immunologists and asthma specialists. We have now, however, reached the advancing edge of research and any ideas of applying this new knowledge to try to treat asthma are still speculative. Clearly, if helper T cells are involved in the production of both allergic asthma (via IgE and mast cells) and non-allergic (via the eosinophils) might it not be possible to treat all kinds of asthma by a suitable attack on the T cells?

This intriguing possibility immediately caused the scientists to think of existing methods of treatment used to prevent the rejection of grafted organs such as kidneys and hearts. The most important drug used for this purpose is *cyclosporin* which acts by disabling T cells. This has been used with great success in transplantation cases since the early 1980s. Trials of small doses of this drug in asthma have actually been carried out on volunteers with long-term severe asthma and the results have been promising. A drug as powerful as cyclosporin has, however, some potentially dangerous side-effects, and it is not thought likely that it will have a permanent place in asthma treatment. Other drugs that interfere with T cells function are in the process of development, however, and some of these may prove suitable. Possible candidates include the experimental drugs FK-506 and rapamycin. You may never hear anything more of these drugs. On the other hand . . . one day they may be as familiar as Ventolin.

A list of the most important drugs currently used to treat asthma

As elsewhere in this book, the trade name for the drug has a capital initial letter. The 'official' or generic name for the drug is given with a lower-case initial letter.

β_2 adrenergic agonists (air tube wideners)

- salbutamol (Aerolin Autohaler, Combivent, Cyclocaps, Salamol, Salbulin, Ventide (with beclomethasone), Ventodisks, Ventolin, Volmax)
- orciprenaline sulphate (Alupent)
- bambuterol (Bambec)
- fenoterol (Berotec 100, Duovent (with ipratropium bromide))
- tolbuterol (Brelomax)
- salmeterol (Serevent)
- terbutaline sulphate (Bricanyl)
- reproterol (Bronchodil)
- pirbuterol (Exirel)
- isoprenaline sulphate (Medihaler-Iso)
- rimiterol (Pulmadil)
- tulobuterol (Respacal).

Corticosteroids (anti-inflammatory drugs)

- beclomethasone (Aerobec Autohaler, Beclazone, Becloforte, Becodisks, Becotide, Filair, Ventide (with salbutamol))
- budesonide (Pulmicort)
- fluticasone propionate (Flixotide).

Xanthine derivatives (air-tube wideners)

- aminophylline (Pecram, Phyllocontin Continus)
- choline theophyllinate (Choledyl)
- theophylline (Franol (with ephedrine hydrochloride), Labophylline, Lasma, Nuelin SA, Slo-Phyllin, Theo-Dur, Uniphyllin Continus).

Anticholinergic drugs (air-tube wideners)

- ipratropium bromide (Antrovent, Duovent (with fenoterol), Ipratropium Steri-Neb)
- oxitropium bromide (Oxivent).

Cromoglycate (mast cell membrane stabilizers)

- sodium cromoglycate (Aerocrom Syncroner, Intal, Intal Syncroner)
- nedocromil sodium (Tilade Syncroner).

Other drugs

- adrenaline (Medihaler-Epi (air-tube widener))
- ephedrine hydrochloride (Cam (decongestant))
- ketotifen (Zaditen (anti-allergic)).

A summary of routine treatment

Remember that everyone with asthma needs regular medical attention. Even if you are convinced that you are getting adequate treatment, you should not try to cope entirely on your own.

Mild or moderate acute attacks

You must be able to judge the severity of your own condition and recognize the need for action. You should understand the effects of different treatments and know the difference between short-term, quick relief drugs which simply combat the immediate narrowing of your bronchial tubes, and longer-acting preventive drugs which reduce the likelihood or severity of attacks. The first you take when required; the second you take systematically and regularly.

You need a plan for coping with a worsening situation and should clearly understand that if an attack doesn't respond to a broncho-dilator inhaler (β_2 receptor agonist), you are in danger and probably require steroids. You must also understand that if, in spite of everything, your asthma is going out of control, you are in an emergency situation and require urgent medical attention, day or night.

By far the best way to take drugs for asthma is by inhalation. This way, they get to the place where they are wanted in the smallest dose needed to produce the desired effect, and with the least chance of causing general upset. Inhalers convert the drug into an aerosol of particles small enough to reach the right place. These may be liquid or a dry powder. Breath-activated powder delivery systems may be easier to use. Lots of asthma patients don't know how to use an inhaler properly. Make sure that you do, because the effective-ness of the treatment depends on it. Read the instructions carefully and follow them exactly or the drug may not get down to the affected bronchial muscles. (See also chapter 8.)

Short-term treatment is by drugs like salbutamol, terbutaline and fenoterol, which stimulate certain of the adrenaline receptors in your air tube muscles and relax them, so widening the air tubes and allowing the air to pass freely.

If attacks go on in spite of this, you need a mast cell membrane stabilizer, such as sodium chromoglycate (Intal) or nedocromil, to stop your mast cells producing substances that are causing your bronchial tubes to go into spasm. These drugs cannot stop an established attack, and only work in cases of allergic asthma. Also, the drug must be present in your body when you encounter the pollens, dust mites, or whatever it is that is causing your asthma. So this is a *long-term* form of treatment. Sodium chromoglycate is inhaled as a powder, from a *Spinhaler* or an aerosol and should be continued for at least several weeks, as directed by your doctor. If Intal fails, you probably need a corticosteroid such as beclomethasone (Becotide) or budesonide (Pulmicort). These, too, are taken by inhaler so as to minimize dosage and general effects.

Salbutamol will usually cope with flare-ups, but severe relapses generally require steroids in larger doses and these must be taken by mouth. So don't delay in consulting your doctor. Above all, you should at all times know about the state of your bronchial tubes. The only way to do this is to use a peak flow rate meter – a simple instrument that measures the peak rates at which you can breathe out. You should be keeping a record of the results, and should know at what point the peak flow rate has become dangerously low (see chapter 6 and 'The peak flow meter plan').

Chronic asthma

'Chronic' simply means 'going on for a long time'. The word comes from the Greek *khronos*, meaning 'time', as in 'chronometer' or 'synchronous'. So although, in a sense, almost all asthma is chronic, the term is used for those cases in which, in the absence of continual treatment, the affected person will be continually inclined to wheeze.

Until fairly recently it was the rule to advise people with chronic asthma to use a β_2 receptor agonist by inhalation four times a day to keep things under control. This, however, means taking a lot of adrenergic drug over a period and there is growing evidence that this is not a very good thing to do. It now seems clear, for reasons that remain obscure, that people who do this are at slightly greater risk of dying from asthma than people who do not. In addition, it is now generally recognized by those who know most about the subject that the basic problem in asthma is concerned as much with inflammation of the lining of the air tubes as with spasm and narrowing of the tubes (see chapter 1).

For these reasons, and as you have already seen, the emphasis has shifted away from β_2 agonists to steroids. The current recommendation is that any person who needs to use β_2 agonists more than once a day should not do so but should rely on inhaled steroids, such as beclomethasone, two puffs twice a day. In those whose asthma is not controlled by this regimen, with or without a β_2 agonist, cromoglycate or ipratropium bromide four times a day should be added.

If this is not enough, further medication in the form of salbutamol may be added. Note that salbutamol and ipratropium taken by inhaler may be less effective than the same drugs taken by a nebulizer (see chapter 8). Salbutamol may also be taken by mouth in a slow-release form such as Volmax. If further treatment is needed, take a xanthine drug by mouth. Slow-release aminophylline is especially useful. But remember that it is all too easy to overdose with xanthine drugs, so start with a small dose and, if necessary, work up.

Severe acute asthma

There is no place for the do-it-yourself treatment of severe, acute asthma, but it is important that you should have an idea of how this is managed. It is also important for you to know how to recognize severe, acute asthma and how vital it is that there should be no delay in the specialist management of this dangerous form of the disease. For these reasons the subject is given a chapter to itself. You can read all about it in chapter 10.

Remember that this is just a summary. You really need to read and master the whole of this book if you are going to become as effective as possible in taking control of your asthma or that of your child. Remember, also, that however much you know about it, asthma management should always be under the control of your doctor.

8
All about inhalers

The use of inhalers – a practice almost unique to asthma – has revolutionized the treatment of this disease. A drug taken by mouth will be distributed throughout the whole body in roughly equal concentration, so that all tissues receive the same dose, whether they need it or not. For the purposes of argument, let us suppose that the bulk of the air tube linings is one thousandth of the bulk of all the tissues of the body. This means that, for a drug taken by mouth, the body must receive one thousand times the total dose needed to produce the desired effect in the air tubes. But if the whole of the drug can be delivered directly to the tube linings, the body will receive that amount and no more.

Looked at in this way it is readily apparent how advantageous it is to use inhalational treatment whenever this is possible. Fortunately, for the enormous majority of people with asthma, inhalational treatment is all that is required. It cannot be denied, however, that, even by the inhalational route, more of the drug is commonly swallowed and absorbed than is delivered directly to the place where it is needed. Nevertheless, inhalation of drugs means that a great deal less must be taken for the same therapeutic effect.

Another advantage of inhaling the required drug is the speed of action achieved. When a drug is taken by mouth it must first take time to pass down through the stomach and into the small intestine. This may take an hour or two, sometimes longer. The drug must then be absorbed through the wall of the intestine into the blood vessels in the wall. It must then pass through the liver where it may be acted on by the liver cells. Only when it reaches the general circulation will it be carried by the blood to the lungs where, in considerable dilution, it reaches the affected parts.

Metered dose aerosol inhalers

The metered dose inhaler is a pressurized device that delivers the correct dose of medication – whether β_2 receptor agonist, anticholinergic agent or steroid (see chapter 7) – through its oral tube. This is not to say that the correct dose actually reaches the air tubes where it is to act. The correct dose will only be achieved if the device is used properly. All asthma patients require instruction in the correct use of inhalers and many take quite a while to acquire the skill needed. Some never do and have to have a different form of treatment.

Here are the essential points:

- Give the canister a good shake. This ensures that the drug is evenly dispersed in the propellant. It also provides reassurance that the canister is not empty.
- Make sure that the canister is held upright in use. If this is not done the internal metering chamber will not refill and the next dose delivered will be inadequate.
- Be quite certain that you are breathing in slowly and steadily at the time you activate the inhaler.
- If you can do it effectively, hold the inhaler so that the mouthpiece is an inch or two away from your open mouth.
- Do not allow the shock of the cold spray to stop this slow, steady inhalation.
- Continue to breathe in fully after the shot of medication and then hold your breath for a count of five to ten seconds.

If your dosage requires two puffs, do not try to deliver both of these during the same inspiration. Just repeat the above routine, holding your breath after each inhalation. If you adopt the inch-from-the-mouth method, do ensure that you are aiming straight, so that everything coming from the inhaler enters your mouth. It's no good if you just spray around your lips.

Insufflators

This is the general term for a class of inhalers that deliver a little cloud of drug in dry powder form. Finely powdered medication works just as well as liquid medication, as the tiny particles quickly dissolve in the layer of fluid that covers all cells. Dry powder is delivered by various devices.

The rotacap system uses capsules that are opened by turning the container. This frees the powder within the device so that it can be inhaled through a fine mesh without inhaling the half capsule. Most of the drugs used to treat asthma are available for delivery from insufflators.

The Spinhaler is a little more complicated. It contains a small internal propeller that rotates under the influence of the inspired airflow. The end of the propeller shaft is hollowed to accommodate a capsule of the drug in powder form. When the outer sliding sleeve is pushed firmly in and out again, spring-loaded spikes pierce the capsule. Rotation of the propeller then drives out the powder by centrifugal force and the powder is carried into the lungs in the inspired air. Like all powder devices, the Spinhaler and its capsules must be kept completely dry.

One advantage of insufflators is that the drug is delivered only when the user inhales through the device. Thus, none of the skills needed for successful use of a metered dose inhaler apply. Quite small children can readily learn to use an insufflator device. Much the same applies to nebulizers (see below) and to metered dose inhalers used in conjunction with large-volume spacers (see below).

Commonly used insufflators include Becotide Rotahaler (beclomethasone), Cyclocaps Cyclohaler (salbutamol), Ventolin Rotahaler (salbutamol) and Intal Spinhaler (cromoglycate).

Nebulizers

A nebulizer is a device for converting a liquid into a cloud of tiny particles. This can be done in various ways. Most nebulizers are just variants of the common paint spray. At one time, nebulizers were to be found on every lady's dressing table in the form of a perfume spray. The principle of this kind of nebulizer is simple. If a high-speed jet of air is directed across the top of a narrow tube, the other end of which is dipped in a liquid, a spray will result. This is because of the venturi effect. The flow of air across the top of the tube causes a drop in the pressure in the upper part of the tube and liquid is sucked up. If the top of the tube is made very narrow a fine jet of liquid emerges which is at once dispersed in small droplets by the high-speed air flow.

In a practical nebulizer the air jet can be obtained from a cylinder of compressed air or oxygen, or from an electric compressor, or even just a simple foot pump. The spray is not directed straight out of the device but is released into a wide chamber so that large liquid particles are retained and only the smallest can escape.

Another kind of nebulizer, using a totally different principle, is the ultrasonic nebulizer. This is also quite simple. The device uses a small, horizontally placed, piezo-electric crystal fed with an alternating current at a frequency much higher than can be heard. A piezo-electric crystal is a flat crystal of quartz, barium titanate or other material with a metal plate deposited on its opposite sides. When an electric current is applied to the plates the crystal twists slightly in one direction; and when the current is reversed, the crystal twists the other way. A high-frequency alternating current thus causes the crystal to vibrate strongly. Lying on top of the diaphragm is a small, open dish into which the medication solution is placed. This too is caused to vibrate and the movement is so vigorous that numerous small particles break out of the liquid and form a mist in the air above the dish. This air is then inhaled. Some specialists suggest that the piezo-electric nebulizers are less satisfactory than the venturi type. It is thought that the kind of mist produced can even, in some cases, trigger off narrowing of the air tubes.

Nebulizers are often fitted with a face mask so as to ensure that, if properly used, all the air breathed contains the medication. Others may have a mouthpiece similar to that on a metered-dose inhaler. Nebulizers have one great advantage over normal inhalers. They are capable of getting the drugs to the air tubes and controlling an attack even if the movement of air in and out of the lungs is markedly reduced. This is because when a nebulizer is used, all the air inhaled over a substantial period of time contains the required medication. Thus, a good nebulizer, properly used, can often terminate an attack that fails to respond to the use of a metered dose inhaler. Nebulizers are widely used both in hospitals and in the home.

Particle size

This is very important because liquid particles larger than a certain size (about 10 μ) never reach the air passages but are simply retained in the mouth or throat. The particle size is largely determined by the speed of the air jet at the venturi, and this, in turn is determined by the flow rate. So a minimum air flow rate is required if the particle size is to be acceptably small. Studies have shown that, ideally, this should not be less than six litres per minute, preferably eight. This rate can readily be achieved by a small electrically driven air compressor, but the normal domestic oxygen cylinders can achieve only half this rate, and will take about 20 minutes to nebulize 4 ml of solution. If adapted to run at the higher rate, they empty very quickly. The large hospital oxygen cylinders can readily supply oxygen at a rate of eight litres per minute.

For these reasons, many asthma patients at home use a nebulizer operated by a foot pump of a type similar to that used, in emergency, to blow up car tyres. If attacks are not too severe the foot pump can be operated by the patient. Otherwise, a second person can do the pumping.

How nebulizers are used

Nebulizers can be used to administer β_2 receptor agonist drugs, especially fenoterol, reproterol, salbutamol and terbutaline; steroids, especially beclomethasone; sodium cromoglycate; and ipratropium bromide. Beta stimulators are especially effective by nebulizer and are said to work as well given in this way as they do when injected intravenously.

The dose of medication to be taken can be diluted to varying degrees. Since some fixed quantity of residual solution is always left in the device, the greater the dilution the less the waste of medication. At the same time, higher dilutions mean that it takes longer to receive the full dose. Check the instructions with your own device, but the chances are that a volume of about 4 ml will be a suitable compromise between economy and duration of treatment.

Children can be helped to use a nebulizer under adult supervision using either a face mask or a mouthpiece. Masks should, however, be held in place and not fixed over the face.

In some cases the expense and trouble of a nebulizer can be avoided by a simple expedient – that of using a large-volume spacer. Other than in particularly severe cases, a spacer is always worth trying.

Large-volume spacers

Spacers are very simple devices that have advantages and benefits far greater than their cheapness and simplicity would suggest. A spacer is simply a clear plastic bottle-like container with a mouthpiece at one end and a hole at the other into which a metered dose inhaler can be fitted. Inside the spacer, near the mouthpiece end, is a one-way valve that allows air to be sucked out of the spacer but prevents air from being blown into it. The volume of the spacer is such that the delivered dose from the inhaler is fully suspended and evenly distributed in the air within the device. The pear-shaped design of the spacer ensures that the minimum amount of the drug is retained on the inner walls of the chamber. This means that no skill or co-ordination is required, and it is sufficient simply to breathe quietly through the mouthpiece.

One of the main reasons why asthma treatment fails is that the medication doesn't get to the place where it is needed. This is usually because the person concerned is not using the inhaler properly. Anything that can make this easier, therefore, is valuable. But this is by no means the only advantage of large-volume spacers. Probably the main advantage is that using a spacer increases the proportion of the dose of medication actually reaching the air tubes, while at the same time reducing the proportion that is absorbed into the bloodstream. This effect has been studied using a radioactive tracer substance. When pressurized aerosol metered dose inhalers are used directly into the mouth, only 10 to 15 per cent of the medication actually reaches the air tubes; the rest is deposited in the mouth and throat and, unless precautions are taken, will be swallowed and absorbed into the body. When a large-volume spacer is used with the same inhalers, 20 per cent of the drug reaches the air passages of the lungs and only 16 per cent is deposited in the mouth and throat. The remainder is retained in the spacer.

Spacer devices with a soft plastic mask attachment are highly effective in delivering medication to young infants. Since no special timing skills are required, they can also be used, without a mask, by children as young as two years old.

Whatever drugs are used, it can be shown by actual clinical trials that treatment is more effective when a large-volume spacer is used. For some of the drugs used to treat asthma, it is of no great consequence if a proportion is absorbed. But now that steroids are being used more extensively it is obviously desirable to try to increase the ratio of drug delivered to the air tubes to that absorbed. This is especially important in cases in which the severity of the disease requires maximal inhaled dosage of steroid.

Several large-volume spacers are in common use today. The Astra Nebuhaler is a one-piece chamber of 750 ml capacity. The Intal Fisonair is a two-piece 700 ml chamber device with a metered dose aerosol delivering 5 mg of sodium cromoglycate per dose. The Aerocrom Synchroner delivers cromoglycate and salbutamol through an integral spacer device. The Volumatic is a two-piece, 750 ml capacity spacer device with a one-way valve and mouthpiece, designed to be used with an aerosol inhaler with actuator. It is suitable for use with Becloforte, Becotide, Flixotide, Serevent, Ventide and Ventolin inhalers.

Small-volume spacers are also readily available and are, of course, much more portable. The Pulmicort spacer, for instance, is a neat, collapsible device that uses a standard inhaler and closes into a space not much larger than a normal inhaler. It has to be said, however, that the small-volume spacer is less efficient and less generally satisfactory than the large-volume spacer.

9

The emotional dimension

There is plenty of evidence that asthma can be greatly affected, both for worse and for better, by emotional and psychological factors. This is hardly surprising. If someone were to take you by the neck and squeeze your windpipe until you were barely able to breathe, and were to maintain the pressure for quarter of an hour, you would certainly experience an emotional reaction.

Research suggests that emotional factors are important in about half the cases of asthma. For many asthmatics and their families this seems obvious. For these, it is a commonplace that emotional upset can and does trigger attacks. Sometimes the influence of such factors is less obvious, however, but may still be very strong, as in the case of Mario Grayson.

CASE HISTORY

Mario was inclined to be sceptical about his mother's suggestions as to the cause of his asthma attacks, but events proved that she was right.

PERSONAL DETAILS

Name: Mario Grayson
Age: 15
Occupation: Schoolboy
Family: Only child. Parents alive and well.

MEDICAL BACKGROUND

Mario has atopic asthma (see chapter 2) and had fairly severe attacks throughout his childhood. Unfortunately, the condition did not clear up at the time of puberty, as hoped. His mother was a nurse, his father is a professional physiologist and they are unusually well informed on the subject of asthma. Various allergens, including house dust mite excreta and tartrazine food colouring, have been identified and, in the main, successfully avoided. There were, however, some other less apparent trigger factors.

THE PRESENT COMPLAINT

After Mario started at a grammar school, his asthma, although still intermittent, seemed to get worse, and his parents became concerned at the rate at which he was getting through beclomethasone (Becotide) and other inhalers. The school authorities were also unhappy and suggested that he needed further medical attention. At the PTA meetings Mario's parents were told that he was a hard-working, conscientious scholar whose results were excellent and who was expected to do well academically. One teacher thought that he might be inclined to worry unduly about his work.

THE CONSULTATION WITH THE FAMILY DOCTOR

Mario, who believes he knows all about asthma, is reluctant to agree to see the family doctor but is finally persuaded to go and see her. He tells the doctor that he is sure that his attacks are caused by something in the school. He says that the school is 'frightfully dusty' and that he is probably inhaling mite droppings or some other allergens.

The doctor, who has discussed the matter privately with Mario's mother, asks him which subjects he finds most difficult. Mario insists that none of them cause him particular problems. Soon, however, the doctor establishes that there is a definite relationship between Mario's biology studies and his asthma attacks. Mario agrees and says that there is probably an allergen in the biology lab – possibly formaldehyde preservative. The doctor confirms that this is a common trigger for asthma, but quickly discovers that Mario's attacks have not been particularly associated with dissections or even with working in the lab. A few more questions show that Mario is very much aware of his father's anxiety that he should become a doctor. This, explains Mario, is the last thing he wants to do. He plans to study English. His only real interest is in English literature and his firm intention is to become a writer.

THE DOCTOR'S COMMENTS

The doctor asks for a report from the school and has a discussion with Mario's parents. Finally, she sees Mario again. She tells him that, as with most cases of asthma, there are probably several factors triggering off attacks. Her enquiries, however, show that in recent months one particular factor has been important –

Mario's conflict between his career wishes, his desire to do well in all subjects, and his dislike of disappointing his father. She tells him that his mother has been keeping a record of his attacks and has shown a close correlation with biology tests and with career interviews. The doctor also says that the report she has had from the school indicates that he has an unusually high aptitude for literature. The career advisor believes that he is better suited to literary studies than to medicine.

Mario says he has been aware of this for years. He asks what all this has to do with his asthma. The doctor explains that mental tension that cannot readily be resolved is liable to cause tightening of the air tubes by way of the vagus nerve. Mario tells her he has known about this for ages. She also explains that the state of the mind can even influence the effectiveness of adrenergic stimuli and drugs. Mario admits that he did not know this. The doctor asks him to think about it.

THE FOLLOW-UP

After a long family discussion, Mario's father assures him that he is not going to dictate the direction of his career. If, by the time he is ready to go to university, he still wants to read English, there will be no objection.

Almost from that day Mario's attacks become markedly less frequent and less severe.

The effect of suggestion

Research has shown that, in some asthmatic people, psychological suggestion can have a remarkable effect both in increasing or in decreasing the severity of asthma. Since the autonomic nervous system is greatly affected by the state of the mind, this should not occasion surprise. Indeed, the surprising thing is that only a proportion of people with asthma seem to be much affected by mental and emotional factors. These studies showed, for instance, that if asthmatic people were told that they were breathing in an aerosol of substances to which they knew themselves to be allergic, they would immediately start wheezing, even if the material was completely bland – just a mist of sterile saline solution. On the other hand, people who were told that they were inhaling an effective asthma medication, but who were actually having the same aerosol, were found to breathe more easily.

For psychologically sensitive asthmatics, emotional stress and the effects of suggestion can be very important. One of the most impressive and influential forms of suggestion is the concern, or even conviction, that one is not going to be able to get enough air. Even for the most mentally hardy and courageous this can be an experience that readily brings on panic. Panic causes tightening of the voluntary muscles and may actually interfere with the full action of the muscles we use to breathe – the voluntary muscles of respiration. These are the intercostal muscles that raise the ribs and swing them outwards, the diaphragm and, when necessary, the muscles in the neck and shoulders that can pull up the collar bones and upper ribs. The latter are called the *accessory muscles of respiration* and, other than during strenuous or athletic activity, you should seldom need to use them.

Obviously, if the air tubes are narrowed by tight and abnormal contraction of the smooth (non-voluntary) muscles in their walls, the voluntary muscles of respiration must work harder to get the necessary air into the lungs. Expiration, which is normally a passive process brought about by the elasticity of the lungs, will also have to become active and involve the voluntary muscles. Thus, any interference with the free action of the voluntary muscles as a result of panic or psychological tension can make things a great deal worse.

The point of all this is that such interference is unnecessary. If people can somehow learn the difficult art of relaxing themselves out of panic, the effects will be that much less severe. The first step is to recognize that abnormal tensing of muscles is occurring. After that, the process is one of systematically letting each group of tensed muscles go slack. To do this in the course of an asthma attack is far from easy, but you will find that you can do it more readily if you practise regularly when you are *not* having an attack.

One way to practise relaxation is to start with your feet and work up. Do the exercise while reclining comfortably in a chair. First, strongly contract the muscles that flex or extend your ankles. Hold this tension for a few seconds and then let it go completely. Then tighten the muscles that bend your knees, but keep your knees unbent. Hold and let go completely. Repeat with thigh and buttock muscles, then with the wrists, elbows and shoulders. The most important part is the total relaxation after each short period of tension. Finally, have one major effort in which all the muscles you have tightened are held for a few seconds in high tension and then completely relaxed so that your whole body is floppy. Once you become good at this you will find that you can cope better with panic tension.

People who deliberately induce asthma attacks

Many people with asthma are well aware that they can bring on an attack at will. This can be done by deliberate, unnecessary coughing or by deliberate hyperventilation – sustained, deep and rapid breathing. Many children know that they can induce an asthmatic attack by crying or by these other means. Some of them use induced asthma as a manipulative weapon to try to control their parents or to avoid school or as a protest against being asked to eat unpopular food. Children have been known systematically to use induced asthmatic attacks to stop their parents from going out in the evening. This is a highly effective ploy, especially with conscientious and concerned parents who are aware that asthma attacks can rapidly worsen and become dangerous. Parents who are aware that their child is inducing attacks must make it unequivocally clear to the child that such behaviour is unacceptable.

Occasionally, manipulative activity of this kind persists into adult life. This is not a mature and dignified way to behave. If you are aware that you are using your asthma as a weapon in a social war you should ask yourself why it is necessary to do this and whether there is a better way of handling the problem. Maybe you need counselling. You should also ask yourself whether the health dangers of the additional and unnecessary attacks are justified by the dubious advantages you gain by them.

10

How severe acute asthma is treated

The management of an unusually severe or prolonged attack of asthma is a job for a doctor, and very severe attacks should always be treated in hospital. Doctors know that asthma can worsen rapidly to the point at which a person's life is in danger. They also know that, if this happens, the patient needs the attention of specialists with experience of dealing with such cases. So if you are in any doubt, call your doctor or an ambulance or get the person concerned to the emergency department of a hospital. It is only in hospital that the full equipment needed to manage dangerous cases is likely to be found. People who die from asthma nearly always do so outside hospital, or are brought in to hospital so late, and in such an advanced stage of oxygen lack, that even the best treatment cannot save them.

So the purpose of this chapter is not to teach you how to treat very severe asthma but to show you how necessary it is in such cases to get the patient to the experts with minimal delay. If you can get a doctor at a reasonably early stage, well and good. Your doctor will know when further medical attention is needed. If you cannot, summon an ambulance and give full details of the severity of the attack. The paramedics of the emergency services know all about the dangers of acute, severe asthma.

Early warning signs

There are some very useful early indications that an acute asthma attack may be imminent. The most important of these is a drop in the peak expiratory flow rate (see chapters 5 and 6). This is, of course, the reason why regular, routine checks with the peak expiratory flow meter are so essential. Other warning suggestions of an acute attack include:

- obvious worsening of asthma symptoms;
- the need for more frequent β_2 receptor agonist (bronchodilator) use;
- failure of normal treatment to have its full usual effect;
- disturbed sleep;

- reduced ability to take exercise;
- a tendency to breathlessness at rest;
- a history of previous severe, acute attacks.

The signs should never be ignored. If you realize that they are danger signs and report them to your doctor, the chances are that a severe, acute attack can be avoided. Unfortunately, some people with asthma are particularly prone to suffer such attacks so that, whatever they do, it is always possible that an attack of severe, acute asthma may occur. In such cases it is not good enough just to wait for an acute, severe attack before doing anything about it. There should be a positive plan of action agreed with the family doctor and the local hospital.

How to recognize severe acute asthma

You are not likely to be in doubt about the diagnosis. All the usual symptoms of an asthmatic attack are present. The breathing is laboured and the wheeze loud, especially on expiration. In spite of the difficulty, the affected person will be trying to breath more rapidly than normal. The chest will be permanently expanded. The victim will be unable to lie down and hardly able to speak. Oxygen lack shows itself by a bluish-purple discoloration of the face, especially the lips and around the mouth. This is called *cyanosis* and it is a most important sign that not enough oxygen is getting through. There is obvious distress. The muscles of the neck and shoulders are being used to try to assist in the breathing. There is sweating and the pulse is racing.

The state of the pulse is an important sign. The fast pulse occurs for three reasons:

- it may simply be a reflection of the patient's anxiety;
- it may be caused by the use of a bronchodilator such as isoprenaline or aminophylline that stimulates the adrenaline receptors;
- it may be due to the need to circulate the blood faster because the body is not getting enough oxygen.

The latter is a serious state of affairs. Since you cannot tell why the pulse rate is high, you must assume the worst.

There is another and even more significant pulse sign. The pulse may become less forceful or even disappear briefly while the patient is breathing in, and then return to normal force during expiration. This sign, known as *pulsus paradoxus*, is an indication that the heart is being compressed. It suggests a severe, acute attack requiring urgent specialist attention.

Any person showing these signs and experiencing these symptoms is in danger and must be got to hospital immediately. This is a medical emergency. It is better to get an ambulance than to drive the patient yourself. Ambulance crew can start emergency treatment, including oxygen by mask, and an ambulance will probably get the victim to hospital quicker than you can. They are also able to radio in details so that the hospital accident and emergency reception staff will be prepared.

Management in hospital

The first stage in the management is essentially the same as you would do yourself – give a β_2 receptor agonist. In hospital, however, this is likely to be given by nebulizer or by injection. Any patient showing signs of oxygen deficiency, such as cyanosis or pulsus paradoxus, will be given warm, humidified oxygen by mask. An intravenous drip will be set up and an infusion of saline or other fluid started. This provides a quick way to get drugs into the body and also ensures that the fluid levels and blood volume are properly maintained.

A chest X-ray may also be taken at this stage, especially if there is any suspicion that the patient might have suffered a collapse of one lung from leakage of air from the lung into the space between the lung and the chest wall. This is called *spontaneous pneumothorax* and can, of course, make matters very much worse for an asthmatic. Spontaneous pneumothorax is hard to diagnose without an X-ray if it occurs in the course of an asthmatic attack.

When β_2 agonists are given by injection, this is done very carefully by an experienced doctor using equipment capable of precise measurement of dosage. This is especially important in children because children's hearts are particularly sensitive to these drugs given in this way. The procedure is usually accompanied by continuous monitoring of the action of the heart by electrocardiography (ECG). If routine β_2 agonists fail, doctors will often try an injection of adrenaline. In such cases, it is more important to get the air passages open than to worry about the side-effects of the drug, even if these are unpleasant.

If there is inadequate or absent response to β_2 agonist drugs, the doctors will want to know the actual levels of oxygen and carbon dioxide in the blood. This is the critical information on which management is based. If oxygen cannot get in properly the oxygen (O_2) levels in the blood will drop. If carbon dioxide cannot get out properly, the carbon dioxide (CO_2) levels in the blood will rise. Blood gas measurement is done by passing a fine tube called a catheter along an artery into one of the main central vessels. This catheter has a special tip capable of monitoring the blood gases and the acidity of the blood. It is, of course, the gas levels in the blood returning from the lungs that is of primary interest. This is why arterial blood must be sampled rather than blood from a vein.

In mild asthma, the arterial blood (plasma) oxygen (PO_2) is normal and the plasma carbon dioxide (PCO_2) is slightly decreased. In moderately severe asthma there is a slight decrease in PO_2 and, because of increased respiratory effort, a moderate decrease in PCO_2. In a severe asthmatic attack there is a moderate decrease in blood oxygen and the PCO_2 is normal. But in very severe asthma the PO_2 drops markedly and the PCO_2 starts to rise. This is a critical sign indicating that fatal respiratory failure may not be far off.

Checks on the blood gases can thus give a precise indication of the degree of airway obstruction and of the level of danger to the patient. A less precise but much simpler method of estimating blood oxygen is the *pulse oximeter* – a simple device that clips onto a finger or earlobe and measures oxygen by the colour change in the blood it causes. Well-oxygenated blood is bright red; blood low in oxygen is a dark purplish colour. This is what causes cyanosis, but the change can also be measured by photoelectric methods.

If, after about an hour, there is no sign of improvement, a large dose of steroid, such as prednisolone, will be given by intravenous injection. Aminophylline may also be given intravenously. Sometimes additional attempts to widen the airways are made in the form of ipratropium bromide inhalation. A constant check is kept on the acidity of the blood. This must be maintained within narrow limits. Deviation from these limits in the form of a rise in acidity will call for infusion of bicarbonate solution. Physiotherapy, in the form of chest percussion to help to bring up sticky lung tube secretions, may improve matters. Patients suffering from a severe asthmatic attack are never given sedatives of any kind. These could be very dangerous as they all tend, to a greater or lesser degree, to diminish respiratory effort. The more powerful sedatives, such as morphine, would probably be fatal.

If the attack persists for more than 24 hours in spite of treatment, and the blood gas analysis shows no rise in the oxygen levels, the doctors may decide that the time has come to resort to a more direct means of getting oxygen into the blood. It is seldom necessary to do so, but if the blood gas checks show a dropping PO_2 and a rising PCO_2 there may be no choice. Indications for this ultimate procedure also include:

- obvious deterioration in the patient's general condition
- drowsiness
- mental confusion
- severe muscular fatigue
- lassitude
- inability to cough
- a lapse into coma.

The final measure involves passing a wide tube through the mouth, over the tongue and down through the voice box (larynx) and into the upper end of the windpipe (trachea). This tube has a balloon section near its tip which can be inflated so as to seal the tube snugly into the trachea. Once in place, the tube is connected to a positive pressure mechanical ventilator that can actually force oxygen into the lungs by sheer pressure.

11
Avoiding asthma

It is obviously far better to avoid asthma attacks, if possible, than to have to treat them. For this reason it is important for you to find out, if you can, what factors bring on an attack. This is especially so in the case of allergic asthma as there are many possible allergens, some of them unexpected. A bit of detective work may sometimes be required, but remember that allergy to most of the common asthma-precipitating substances can be proved by a simple skin prick test. From your point of view there is very little to this test. Single drops of solutions of the common allergens are laid out in neat rows on your arm, or elsewhere on your skin, and given an identifying mark. Needles are then used to prick the skin lightly through each drop. After about 15 minutes there will be a definite red reaction at any site at which an allergen to which you are sensitive was present.

No list of allergens is ever likely to be complete, but some allergens are much commoner than others, and the following reminder list contains most of them:

- household dust mite products, especially mite excreta
- cockroach excreta
- insect parts
- silverfish
- dust lice
- domestic animal skin flakes (dander)
- animal fur
- cat saliva
- pigeon droppings
- budgerigar droppings
- tree pollen grains
- grass pollen grains
- fungus spores
- organic fibres and lint
- pyrethrum insecticide
- orris root
- coffee bean dusts
- soya bean products

- flax seed
- cotton seed
- vegetable gums
- bee, wasp and other insect stings
- numerous industrial chemicals.

It is well worth checking through this list. It may bring to your notice possible allergens you may not have considered.

Once you have the triggers that are bringing on your attacks, you must of course try to avoid them. This is often more easily said than done, but, apart from the avoidance of attacks, it is important because the more frequent the exposure to the allergen, the worse the asthma is likely to get. This is because repeated exposure to allergens increases the amount of IgE, as well as the number of mast cells and eosinophils, in the body.

Keeping away from the allergen

It is only when you know the identity of the allergen that you can intelligently plan a strategy for avoidance. It is unlikely that you will be able to avoid the allergen altogether, but you can do a great deal to reduce the number of attacks.

What to do about house dust mites

Regular hoovering is less effective than most people realize. A thorough vacuum clean can immediately reduce the mite population by 70 per cent, but these little creatures breed very rapidly and the population will return to the previous level within a week. Dust mite excreta are highly allergenic and are an important cause of repeated asthma attacks. Remember that vacuuming causes mite faeces to become airborne, so the cleaning should never be done by the asthma victim. Asthma sufferers must keep out of any rooms that are being cleaned.

Some vacuum cleaner bags allow allergen particles to get through. Tough, disposable paper bags are more efficient than the earlier type of cloth bags that have to be emptied, but neither can be completely relied on. Particles are more likely to be trapped if the bag has already been used for a while so that the air has to pass through a thick layer of fluff and dust.

Miticides are chemicals that can kill house dust mites, and are worth considering. They include tannic acid, crotamiton and benzyl benzoate. Some people treat their carpets with these. Unfortunately, benzyl benzoate can cause severe skin irritation and may damage the eyes. So you must be careful not to overdo the use of these miticide substances. Probably the most effective measure against mites is to deprive them of their favourite habitat – cotton or linen sheets, pillow-slips, duvet covers and mattresses. If these are enclosed in polythene or nylon bags the mites will have a hard time of it. Do be very careful, however, with children's bedding, to ensure that there is no possibility of a plastic bag coming loose and causing suffocation. Bedding should also be washed frequently at a high temperature setting of the washing machine. This will help to keep down the mite population.

Children's soft toys are also common breeding grounds for house dust mites. Teddy bears, given to comfort distressed asthmatic children, can soon become unsuspected causes of perpetuating the problem. The best solution, in this case is a weekly stay in the freezer. This can be relied on to kill any mites present.

House dust mites are also very sensitive to reduced atmospheric humidity. Experience has shown that people with severe allergic asthma are often greatly improved during a spell in an Alpine region at an altitude above 1,000 metres. At such altitudes, the air is so dry that mites cannot survive.

Domestic animals

This is a difficult and emotive subject, especially if children are involved. There is, unfortunately, no doubt that animal dander, hair, urine and saliva can all be potent allergens that can trigger asthmatic attacks. Cats seem to be the greatest source of trouble, but dogs, birds, small rodents such as hamsters, and horses can all be the source of allergens that cause asthma. At the same time it has to be recognized that many children are emotionally dependent on their animals and would suffer severely if forcibly deprived of them. It is even possible that to do so would be to make the asthma worse.

These facts make decisions difficult. Existing, much-loved, pets should certainly not be disposed of without clear evidence that they are actually causing asthma. You would be justified, in such cases, in asking for a specific RAST test for IgE to prove that the animal was responsible. RAST is an abbreviation for *radio-allergo-sorbent test*, a test that can actually determine the specific form of IgE that the patient is producing and thus identify the allergen. Even if the test is positive, however, this is no indication that the animal is the sole trigger for asthmatic attacks. Getting rid of it will not necessarily improve matters.

If there is a proposal to acquire a new animal pet in a household with an asthma sufferer, the matter is easier – forget it. People with asthma may not be allergic to any animal but daily exposure to a domestic animal is likely to bring about a new allergy to an animal product within a matter of weeks and this will almost certainly make the asthma worse.

Pollens and spores

Seasonal allergens such as pollens and fungal spores are not of primary importance in asthma, although they very commonly trigger off attacks in asthmatics who also suffer from other causes. Some people with asthma suffer wheezing attacks only on exposure to seasonal allergens, but in such cases the attacks are seldom very serious.

The exposure to pollens and spores during the periods of high pollen count can be reduced by some obvious methods such as:

- staying indoors;
- keeping windows closed, even upper-floor windows in tall buildings;
- keeping car windows closed during country trips;
- observing areas of high pollen count;
- avoiding parks and other open spaces with vegetation;
- keeping away from barns, grass-mowing, haymaking;
- wearing a mask over the nose and mouth.

It is not much use tying a handkerchief over the nose and mouths as the pollen grain size is much less than that of the spaces between the threads. Multi-layer masks are more useful, or you might, in extreme cases, resort to a kind of spaceperson's plastic helmet with a wide, flexible tube connected to a portable, battery-powered filter unit on a belt. Units of this kind can certainly eliminate allergens but they can be uncomfortably warm and conspicuous and are inclined to mist up.

Indoors, you can use electrostatic particle precipitators and high-efficiency air-conditioning systems with particle-trapping filters. These are major and expensive items. The domestic 'ionizers' commonly sold for claimed health purposes are not likely to make any difference. Even the best particle precipitators cannot be relied on to deal with heavy particles such as house dust mite excreta. These pass briefly into the air when mattresses, bedding etc. are disturbed and may be inhaled. But they soon settle again and are not removed by air filters.

Avoiding drugs that could precipitate asthma

One of the most important groups of possible triggers for asthma are the drugs. One class of drugs – the beta-blockers – is liable to cause severe attacks in *any* asthmatic person. Other groups of drugs may also cause trouble to asthmatics either by their inherent action or because there happens to be a particular sensitivity to that type of drug.

Beta-blockers

You must be particularly careful to avoid drugs of the β_2 *antagonist* (beta-blocker) class. These drugs are very dangerous for asthmatics as they interfere with the body's normal autonomic system (sympathetic) action in widening the air passages. Beta-blockers may be invaluable to many non-asthmatic people with angina, high blood pressure, heart irregularity, recent heart attacks or severe stress reactions, but they are disastrous for people with asthma. Remember that one of your most valuable groups of drugs are the beta receptor *agonists*. So the last thing you need are beta receptor *antagonists* – which have exactly the opposite effect. In asthma, beta-blockers can threaten life.

You can usually spot a beta-blocker *generic* name by the ending '-olol'. But most people know these drugs by their trade names. Here is a short list of those most commonly used, with the trade names in brackets:

- propranolol (Inderal LA, Beta-Prograne)
- atenolol (Beta-Adalat, Tenormin, Tenif, Totamol)
- labetalol (Trandate)
- oxprenolol (Trasicor, Slow-Trasicor)
- acebutolol (Sectral)
- timolol (Blocardren, Betim, Timoptol)
- metoprolol (Betaloc, Lopressor)
- sotalol (Beta-Cardone, Sotacor)
- esmolol (Brevibloc)
- nadolol (Corgard)

- bisoprolol (Emcor, Monocor)
- pindolol (Visken).

Not all beta-blockers are equally dangerous. Some are claimed to be highly selective for the β_1 receptors rather than the β_2 receptors. High selectivity may not be enough, however, and you should remember that *all* beta-blockers have some action in blocking the β_2 receptors. So, unless the risk of not using any type of beta-blocker drug is considerable, you should avoid them all. This, of course, is a decision for your doctor, who will take all factors into consideration. But it must be uncommon for any known asthmatic person to be deliberately prescribed a beta-blocker drug, except, perhaps, in the form of eye drops. Even these could be dangerous. *Non-selective* beta-blockers (β_1 and β_2 antagonists) should *never* be used. If you *have* to use selective β_1 antagonist beta-blockers, do so with great care and watch out for any signs of an asthma attack.

Cholinergic drugs

These drugs are used to treat various conditions including retention of urine, glaucoma and myasthenia gravis. People with asthma should be particularly careful with the following:

- bethanechol (Myotonine)
- neostigmine (Prostigmin)
- distigmine bromide (Ubretid)
- carbachol (Isopto carbachol)
- pilocarpine (Isopto carpine, Minims pilocarpine, Sno Pilo)
- pyridostigmine (Mestinon).

These drugs are not widely used, and several of them only occur commonly in the form of eye drops. Even so, it pays to be careful. Eye drops run down the tear ducts into the nose and can then be absorbed into the bloodstream.

Aspirin and aspirin-like drugs

Sensitivity to aspirin, in that it can trigger an asthmatic attack, is not an allergy in the normal sense of the word. Indeed, this problem does not appear to involve the immune system at all. For that reason, aspirin sensitivity is usually described as a *pseudo-allergy*. From your point of view this fact is entirely academic. The effects are the same.

If you have the slightest suspicion that you have aspirin sensitivity, avoid all forms of aspirin and all aspirin-containing remedies. Remember how many popular medicines contain aspirin. Here is a list of some of these:

- Anadin
- Anadin Extra
- Angettes
- Aspav
- Aspro
- Aspro Clear
- Asprodeine
- Beecham's Powders
- Beecham's Tablets
- Benorylate
- Caprin
- Codiphen
- Codis
- Decrin
- Disalcid
- Disprin
- Disprin CV
- Disprin Extra
- Doxolene Co
- Ecotrin
- Equagesic
- Migravess
- Nu-seals
- postMI 300
- Robaxisal forte
- Solcode
- Solprin
- Veganin
- Vincent's powders
- Winsprin.

Aspirin is acetyl salicylic acid. So any drug containing salicylate of any kind is equally likely to affect you. Remember also that if you are sensitive to aspirin, there is a distinct possibility that you may also be sensitive to any of the range of non-steroidal anti-inflammatory drugs such as:

- aloxiprin (Palaprin forte)
- diclofenac (Voltarol)
- diflunisal (Dolobid)
- fenbufen (Lederfen)
- fenoprofen (Progesic)
- ibuprofen (Brufen)
- indomethacin (Indocid)
- mefenamic acid (Ponstan)
- naproxen (Naprosyn)
- phenylbutazone (Butazolidin)
- piroxicam (Feldene)
- tolmetin (Tolectin).

One thing to remember about drugs is that they need not be consciously taken to have their effects. It is possible to have a severe allergic response from inhaling the fine dust that can arise from a bottle of tablets. People working with drugs in an industrial setting are particularly prone to this unexpected hazard.

Food additives

You may also be sensitive to some commonly used food colouring agents, especially the yellow dye tartrazine. About 50 per cent of all aspirin-sensitive asthmatics are also sensitive to tartrazine. Check for this colorant and other food additives (shown by the letter E followed by a number) in the contents list of any foods you may suspect of triggering an attack. Here are some other additives – colourings, preservatives and antioxidants – that have been found to cause asthma:

- tartrazine (E102)
- quinoline yellow (E104)
- sunset yellow (E110)
- carmoisine (E122)
- amaranth (E123)
- indigo carmine (E132)
- green S (E142)
- annatto (E160b)
- benzoates (E210–219)
- sodium metabisulphite (E223)
- butylated hydroxyanisole (BHA antioxidant) (E320)
- butylated hydroxytoluene (BHT antioxidant) (E321).

Chest infection

If you know that you are prone to asthma attacks whenever you get a cold or a sore throat or an attack of bronchitis you should discuss with your doctor whether respiratory infection prevention is justified. Many doctors would agree that asthmatic people in this category should be given a supply of an antibiotic to be used at the first sign of a respiratory system infection.

Colds and influenza are, of course, caused by viruses and these are quite unaffected by antibiotics. But many colds and cases of 'flu also feature secondary infection with bacteria that *are* susceptible to antibiotics. A great many cases of throat infection, bronchitis and pneumonia are also caused by bacteria that can be killed by antibiotics. Any suggestion of an infection of the bronchi or lungs certainly calls for energetic and early treatment.

Influenza can be a potent trigger of asthma and should be avoided if at all possible. People with asthma should thus ensure that their immunization status is up-to-date. Unfortunately, the viruses that cause influenza change from time to time, sometimes from season to season. So you should get advice on this point from your doctor as each winter approaches.

Other things to avoid

Smoking

Smoking is probably the most dangerous activity in which any person, asthmatic or not, can engage. It is particularly dangerous for asthmatics and nothing can ever justify it. If you are a smoker, the most valuable thing you can do for yourself is to stop right now. Permanently. There is only one way to do this. Get rid of your cigarettes, ash trays, lighter. Forget about nicotine chewing gum, nicotine patches, hypnotism, evening classes on quitting and all the other delaying excuses. Just stop, and never even consider doing it again. That is by far the easiest way. And it is much easier than you think. It is really a choice between sanity and self-indulgence.

Passive smoking

This is less easy to control, but you are perfectly entitled to stand up for your rights to clean air. You will probably have to avoid some places, like pubs, where your rights are likely to be ignored. You can certainly insist on clean air in your home. If necessary, you must make it a moral issue. Fortunately, there is growing recognition of the rights of non-smokers in places of employment and in public places generally.

Atmospheric pollution

Motor vehicle exhaust emission, even in low concentration, is damaging to you. If you can smell exhaust, the levels of nitrogen oxides are certainly above the danger threshold. The situation is worst in bright sunshine and when atmospheric temperature inversion (cold below, hotter above) prevents pollutants rising by normal convection. Sunlight converts the oxygen in nitrogen oxides to the more dangerous ozone. If you live in a busy town, try to avoid the areas of maximum traffic density. When driving, try to choose your routes to minimize exposure to heavy traffic in built-up areas. All this is admittedly difficult, and you are likely to be influenced more by economic than by health considerations. But do try to give sufficient weight to the latter. You only have one life to live and you should do what you can to improve its quality. There are still plenty of rural areas where the air is clean and the surroundings pleasant. Advances in technology are steadily making it more practicable for people to hold down good jobs without necessarily living in towns. Soon teleworking villages will be common. Maybe you can help to promote this excellent idea.

Betel-nut chewing

The betel-nut *Areca catechu*, popular with many Asian people, contains a cholinergic alkaloid called *arecoline*. This statement should be enough to indicate that betel-nut offers potential risks to anyone with asthma. Sure enough, tests have shown that this alkaloid causes a dose-related contraction of the smooth muscle of the bronchial air tubes with narrowing of the tubes whether you suffer from asthma or not. There have been reports of betel-nut chewing immediately before attacks of acute, severe asthma. It may also be significant that in Britain the rate of hospital admissions for severe asthma is higher for Asians than for other groups.

Some asthmatic devotees of the betel-nut appear relatively unaffected by the habit, but even in these it is likely that the peak expiratory rate will be reduced after chewing.

Occupational problems

In chapter 3 – 'Allergy and occupation' – you will find a useful list of the commonest and most dangerous allergens causing industrial asthma. Health and safety regulations do much to reduce the risks of work-related asthma, but these regulations are not always as carefully observed as they should be. This is not necessarily the fault of the employers. Some of these regulations are irksome and unpopular with workers. Nevertheless, you owe it to yourself to ensure that your health does not suffer as a result of your work.

About exercise

Unfortunately, exercise is a potent trigger of asthmatic attacks. The reasons for this are now well known (see chapter 3 – 'Exercise and asthma'), and if you understand them, you will be able to do much to avoid unnecessary attacks. This does not mean avoiding exercise, but it does mean choosing your exercise wisely and ensuring that your air passages – which must pass far more air during exercise than when you are at rest – are fully widened by the use of bronchodilators before you start. And if you are not a swimmer, now might be the time to take it up.

12
Glossary

Acetylcholine An important nerve activator (neurotransmitter) that acts at nerve junctions and at the junctions between nerves and muscles (synapses) to pass on nerve impulses. Various drugs with potential uses in asthma interfere with the action of acetylcholine. See also **anticholinergic drugs**.

Acute Short, sharp and quickly over. Acute conditions usually start abruptly, last for a few days and then either settle or become persistent and long-lasting (chronic). Acute, severe asthma is a dangerous condition formerly known as *status asthmaticus*. From the Latin *acutus*, sharp.

Adrenaline A hormone secreted by the inner part of the adrenal glands. It is produced when unusual efforts are required. It speeds up the heart, widens the air passages, increases the rate and ease of breathing, raises the blood pressure, deflects blood from the intestines to the muscles, mobilizes the body fuel glucose and causes a sense of alertness and excitement. It has been described as the hormone of 'fright, fight or flight'. Adrenaline is available for use as a drug and can be given by injection in asthmatic and allergic emergencies. Because of its widespread and unpleasant effects it is not used for routine asthma treatment. It is also known, especially in the USA, as epinephrine.

Adrenoreceptor One of the many receptor sites on the surface of cells (cell membranes) at which adrenaline and other hormones act to cause muscle to contract or relax. Beta-adrenoceptors occur in the walls of the air tubes of the lungs (bronchi), in blood vessels, the heart, the intestines, the bladder, the womb and elsewhere. Stimulation of these sites in the air tubes causes the tubes to widen. The effect of the hormones at these sites can be promoted by beta-adrenergic **agonists** and prevented by beta-blocker drugs (antagonists).

Aeroallergens Substances that can promote an allergic reaction (**allergens**) and that are carried by moving air. They include tree and grass pollen grains, fungal spores and house dust mite faeces. Aeroallergens are common triggers of asthmatic attacks.

Agonist Any substance or drug that acts at a cell receptor site to produce the same effect as the appropriate normal body's chemical messenger (hormone). Many agonist drugs closely resemble the natural physiological agonists.

Allergen Any substance capable of stimulating the body's immune system into bringing about an allergic reaction in a sensitive person. See also **allergy**.

Allergy Hypersensitivity to body contact with a foreign substance (an **allergen**), especially grass or tree pollens, foods, dust, mites or certain metals such as nickel. The effect may take several forms, including asthma, hay fever, skin weals (urticaria) or eczema (dermatitis). An allergic response implies that there has been a prior contact with the allergen during which the immunological processes leading to the hypersensitivity have occurred. Susceptibility to allergy is often of genetic origin, and is then known as **atopy**. The term allergy derives from the Greek *allos*, other and *ergon*, work.

Alveolus One of the many million tiny, thin-walled air sacs in the lungs, through the walls of which oxygen passes from the air into the blood and carbon dioxide passes out.

Antagonist A drug that counteracts or neutralizes the action of another drug or of a natural body chemical messenger (hormone).

Antibody A protective protein substance, called an immunoglobulin, produced by the B group of lymphocytes (B cells) in response to the presence of a foreign substance (antigen). Antibodies act mainly to immobilize infective organisms and render them susceptible to destruction by phagocytes in the body. In allergic asthma, certain antibodies of the E class (immunoglobulin E or IgE) are intimately involved in the process of triggering the asthmatic attack (see chapter 2).

Anticholinergic drugs Drugs that interfere with the action of **acetylcholine**. They include atropine and atropine-like substances, but the only practical anticholinergic drugs for use in asthma are ipratropium bromide and oxitropium.

Antihistamine drugs See **histamine**.

Atopy An inherited state with related environmental factors that features a **hypersensitivity** reaction associated with immunoglobulin E (IgE). It causes a proneness to asthma, hay fever and eczema (atopic dermatitis). Many cases of atopy are caused by an abnormal gene on chromosome 11 but it seems likely that other abnormal genes are involved. The term is derived from the Greek *a*, 'not' and *topos*, 'a place', in recognition of the fact that the reaction may occur at a different site from that of contact with the causal allergen. Research into atopy has thrown much light on the causation of asthma.

Autonomic nervous system The part of the nervous system that controls unconscious functions, such as the heart beat, the secretion of glands and the contraction of muscles in the walls of blood vessels and the air tubes of the lungs. It is subdivided into the sympathetic and the parasympathetic divisions which are, in general, antagonistic and in balance. The relevance to asthma is that the state of contraction of the muscles in the walls of the air tubes – and hence their bore – is under the control of the autonomic nervous system. Drugs used to treat asthma modify the function of this system either by promoting sympathetic action or blocking parasympathetic action. The term autonomic derives from the Greek *autos*, self, and *nomos*, a law.

Beclomethasone Currently the commonest corticosteroid drug used in the form of an aerosol spray to relieve the symptoms of asthma. Trade names are Aerobec, Beclazone, Becloforte, Becodisks, Beconase, Becotide and Filair.

Benzopyrone A chemical substance related to the vanilla-scented anticoagulant and flavouring agent coumarin. The drug cromoglycate, much used to treat asthma, is a benzopyrone. Benzopyrones are also known as cromones.

Beta$_2$ (β_2) adrenoreceptor agonists The important group of drugs that stimulate certain adrenaline receptors in the muscle cells of the air tubes of the lungs, causing them to widen. As a group, these drugs are known as bronchodilators.

Beta-adrenoceptor blocking drugs Beta-blockers. Drugs that selectively block the action of adrenaline on the beta-adrenoceptors. Beta adrenoceptor stimulation by agonist drugs widens the air tubes; beta-blockers have the opposite effect and are thus dangerous to anyone with asthma.

Bronchus A breathing air tube of the lungs, a branch of the windpipe (trachea) or of another bronchus. The trachea divides into two main bronchi, one for each lung, and these in turn divide into further, smaller bronchi. See also **bronchiole**.

Bronchiole One of the many thin-walled, tubular branches of the bronchi, which extend the airway to the terminal air sacs, the **alveoli**. Bronchi have cartilaginous rings, bronchioles do not.

Candidiasis Infection with the common fungus of the genus candida, especially by the species *candida albicans*. Thrush mainly affects the warm, moist areas of the body such as the mouth or the vagina but any part of the skin may be affected. In asthma, the use of steroid inhalers encourages candidiasis of the mouth and throat. This is minimized if a little water is drunk after using the inhaler. In established candidiasis there is a persistent itching or soreness and characteristic white patches, like soft cheese, with raw-looking inflamed areas in between. The condition is treated with antifungal drugs, such as clotrimazole, miconazole or nystatin.

Capillary The smallest and most numerous of all the blood vessels. Capillaries form dense networks between the arteries and the veins, and it is only in the capillary beds that interchange of oxygen, carbon dioxide and nutrients can take place with the cells.

Cartilage Gristle. A dense form of connective tissue performing various functions in the body such as providing bearing surfaces in the joints, flexible linkages for the ribs, and a supportive tissue in which bone may be formed during growth. The larger air tubes – the trachea and bronchi – are kept open by incomplete rings of cartilage.

Cholinergic Relating to nerves that release **acetylcholine** at their endings, including the nerves to the voluntary muscles and all the parasympathetic nerves supplying the air tubes of the lungs. The term is also used to refer to anything that has effects similar to those of acetylcholine.

Chromosome 11 The chromosome which carries at least one of the genes for the abnormal protein receptor on mast cells. Cells with this abnormal receptor degranulate readily when an allergen such as a pollen grain locks on to IgE antibodies attached to the receptor. The condition of a person who carries this gene is called **atopy.**

Chronic Lasting for a long time. A chronic disorder may be mild or severe but will usually involve some long-term or permanent organic change in the body.

Cilia The microscopic hairlike processes extending from the surface of the cells lining the air tubes of the lungs (*ciliated epithelium*). Cilia perform a synchronized rhythmical lashing motion in such a way as to carry unwanted material out of the air tubes.

Corticosteroids Drugs identical to, or that simulate the actions of, the natural steroid hormones of the outer zone (cortex) of the adrenal glands. Modern synthetic steroids are often many times more powerful than the natural hormones hydrocortisone and corticosterone. They include prednisolone, methylprednisolone, beclomethasone, triamcinolone, dexamethasone, betamethasone, deoxycortone and fludrocortisone.

Cromone See **benzopyrone**.

Degranulation The release from a **mast cell** or an **eosinophil cell** of their granules of **histamine, prostaglandins, leukotrienes**, heparin etc. These are the substances that trigger off an asthmatic attack in the case of allergic asthma (mast cells) and non-allergic asthma (eosinophils). Degranulation of mast cells occurs when the allergen bridges across adjacent IgE molecules (see chapter 2).

Dermatophagoides pteronyssinus The common house dust mite in the United Kingdom. When it was first proved that *D. pteronyssinus* was a cause of asthma, it was assumed that the allergen was part of the mite body. Later it was discovered that the allergen was limited to the mite faeces. Finally, it was established that the allergen was a coating of digestive enzyme surrounding the tiny balls of faeces – the protein-splitting enzyme used by the mite to break down the human skin scales on which it lives.

Dermatophagoides farinae The commonest mite allergen in the USA. See also **Dermatophagoides pteronyssinus**, which it closely resembles.

Diaphragm The dome-shaped muscular and tendinous partition that separates the cavity of the chest from the cavity of the abdomen. When the diaphragm muscle contracts the dome flattens, thereby increasing the volume of the chest, so that air is forced in by atmospheric pressure. In an asthmatic attack the inflow and outflow of air is impeded to a variable degree by narrowing of the air tubes.

Eosinophil A white blood and tissue cell (*leukocyte*) that readily stains with the dye eosin to reveal many red-coloured granules. The eosinophil has long been known to have some connection with allergies and with worm infestation, but its relationship to asthma has only recently been elucidated.

Eosinophilia An increase in the number of **eosinophil** cells in the blood or in the lungs (pulmonary eosinophilia). Eosinophilia is characteristic of asthma, worm infestation, reactions to certain drugs and various allergic conditions (see also chapters 2 and 7).

Ephedrine A drug with a similar action to adrenaline but with a more stimulant effect on the nervous system, causing tremor, anxiety, insomnia and undue alertness. It is sometimes used to treat asthma and other local allergic conditions. Ephedrine nasal drops decongest a swollen nose lining.

Extrinsic Extraneous to a body or system. Originating from outside. For many years, asthma has been almost universally divided into two classes – extrinsic and intrinsic. Extrinsic asthma was deemed to be that triggered by allergens from outside the body, such as pollen grains and house dust mite excreta. Intrinsic asthma was that which appeared to be unrelated to environmental triggers. As knowledge has grown of the true nature of 'non-allergic' asthma and of the role played in it by various environmental irritants, this classification is falling into disuse.

Globulins A group of blood proteins that include the family of immunoglobulins (Ig) or antibodies; the antihaemophilia globulin; antilymphocytic globulin; thyroxine-binding globulin; vitamin D-binding globulin; and many others. In the context of asthma, the immunoglobulin class E (IgE) currently appears to be by far the most important.

Goblet cells The simplest of all the glands of the body. Goblet cells are single, swollen, cuboidal cells that secrete mucus. They are found in large numbers in the single-layered epithelial lining of the air passages of the lungs. In asthma, goblet cells are over-stimulated into producing more than the normal amount of mucus. This contributes to the problem of air tube obstruction. See also **cilia**.

Haemoglobin The iron-containing protein that fills red blood cells. Haemoglobin combines readily but loosely with oxygen in conditions of high oxygen concentration, as in the lungs, and releases it when in an environment low in oxygen, as in the body tissues. In health, each 100 ml of blood contains 12 to 18 g of haemoglobin.

Helper T cells One of the classes of T lymphocytes. The principal function of helper T cells is to provide essential assistance to B lymphocytes (B cells) in the process of producing antibodies. The absence of helper T cells, as in AIDS, results in the inability of the immune system to protect the body against infection. Recent research has shown that helper T cells are involved in the processes of producing 'non-allergic' ('intrinsic') asthma (see chapter 7 – section on advances in treatment).

Histamine A highly biologically active substance found widely in nature. Histamine is one of the main constituents of the granules of **mast cells** and is released when these cells degranulate. Among several actions, it is a potent tightener of the muscles in the air tube walls. Contraction of these muscles narrows the air passages. Antihistamine drugs closely resemble histamine in chemical structure. They occupy and block the receptor sites on cell membranes at which histamine acts, but do not promote its effects. Unfortunately, although antihistamines are very useful in the other respiratory tract mast-cell mediated condition, hay fever, they have no part to play in the treatment of asthma. Indeed, the common central nervous system sedating effect of antihistamines could be dangerous in an asthmatic attack.

House dust mite See **Dermatophagoides pteronyssinus** and **Dermatophagoides farinae**.

Hypersensitivity The state of an allergic person which results from previous exposure to an **allergen** and the production of specific IgE antibodies to that allergen. If the same allergen contacts that person again, there is likely to be almost immediate **degranulation** of **mast cells** and an allergic attack. See also chapter 2.

Idiopathic Of unknown cause. Personal, individual, originating within oneself, without known or obvious external cause.

Immune system The body system of cells that confers the ability to resist infection or the effects of any toxic or dangerous substance. The system operates as a result of prior infection or immunization or the passive transfer of antibodies from the mother across the placenta or in the breast milk. **Hypersensitivity**, which is a feature of anomalous functioning of the immune system, is the cause of the majority of cases of asthma.

Immunoglobulins Antibodies – protective proteins produced by cloned B lymphocyte-derived plasma cells. There are five classes of immunoglobulins, the most prevalent being immunoglobulin G (IgG), or gamma globulin which provides the body's main defence against bacteria, viruses and toxins. Immunoglobulin E (IgE) is the one involved in allergic reactions such as asthma (see chapter 2).

Interleukin-5 A highly active soluble protein substance produced by T cells. Interleukin-5 has been called the B cell growth factor because of its power of stimulating antibody-producing B cells. Its importance in asthma is that it stimulates the production of **eosinophil** cells and prompts their **degranulation**, thereby bringing about attacks of non-allergic asthma.

Intrinsic See **extrinsic**.

Ipratropium bromide A drug with relaxing effects on the air tube muscles similar to those of atropine (Belladonna) but without the undesirable side effects on the nervous system and the activity of the **cilia**. Ipratropium is sold under various trade names such as Atrovent, Ipratropium Steri-Neb, Rinatec, Combivent and Duovent. In the latter two cases, the drug is combined with salbutamol and fenoterol, respectively. See also Chapter 7.

Large-volume spacer A device used in conjunction with an inhaler to disperse the medication more or less evenly in a large volume of air so that this can then be inhaled. The main advantage is that a larger proportion of the drug is carried to the point of action and less deposited in the mouth and throat. The spacer is also helpful to people and children who have difficulty in achieving correct timing with a directly used inhaler. The disadvantages of the large-volume spacer is its considerable bulk in comparison with an inhaler.

Leukotrienes A group of active substances related to **prostaglandins** which are formed in, and released from, damaged cells membranes and pass into the bloodstream. In asthma, leukotrienes are released when **mast cells** are **degranulated**. They cause the muscle in the walls of the air tubes to tighten and small blood vessels to leak fluid and cause local swelling. Some leukotrienes have a powerful effect in attracting cells such as **eosinophils** to the site of their release.

Mast cell The principal culprit in causing the effects of an asthmatic attack in allergic (atopic) asthma. This cell contains granules of highly irritating substances that are released when adjacent antibodies of class IgE attached to the cell membrane are bridged by the **allergen**. These released substances cause the local changes in the air tubes characteristic of an asthmatic attack. The mast cell membrane contains many protein receptors for IgE and recent research has shown that abnormalities in these receptors result from the abnormal gene or genes on chromosome 11 that seem to be the cause of **atopy**.

Metered dose aerosol inhaler The commonest type of inhaler used to treat asthma. Metered dose inhaler containers have a small, subsidiary internal chamber which fills with the liquid medication after each usage. Assuming the container is not empty and that the device is held vertically in use, this ensures that the next delivery will be of the correct amount. Some people find metered dose inhalers difficult to use because of the necessity to time the inhalation properly (see chapter 8) and to continue to inhale while spraying. At best, only about 10 per cent of the dose from a metered dose inhaler reaches the site of the trouble. The remainder is deposited in the mouth and throat and is usually swallowed. These disadvantages can be partly overcome by the use of a **large-volume spacer**.

Nebulizer A device, operated by compressed air or oxygen or by an electric pump or foot pump, for delivering a fine-particle aerosol of asthma medication, over a period, from a dilute solution of the drug. Nebulizers have the advantage over other systems of drug delivery that they can carry medication to the site of the trouble even if the airflow in and out of the lungs is greatly reduced. Their main disadvantage is bulk and expense. See also chapter 8.

Passive smoking Inhaling cigarette smoke exhaled into the local atmosphere by others. Even small quantities of cigarette smoke in the inhaled air can be detrimental to asthmatics. Passive smoking causes a rise in the IgE levels in the bodies of those exposed to it. It has also been shown, incidentally, that the rate of lung cancer in non-smokers rises significantly if they are regularly exposed to other people's cigarette smoke. At least ten separate studies have shown an increase of up to 30 per cent in the risk of lung cancer among non-smokers living with smokers, compared with non-smokers living with non-smokers.

Peak expiratory volume The maximum volume of air that can be breathed out after a maximal indrawing of air. Measurement of this can give valuable information about the state of the air passages in asthma, but it requires bulky and expensive equipment. Because of this, a related parameter, the **peak expiratory flow rate**, is much more commonly assessed. This can be done using a cheap and portable piece of equipment, the **peak expiratory flow meter**.

Peak expiratory flow rate A test widely used to determine the presence, and assess the degree, of any kind of obstruction to the air passages. The method is especially valuable in the assessment of asthma and of the response to treatment.

Peak expiratory flow meter A simple device, available in various design forms, that provides a numerical measure of the maximum achievable rate of flow of the expired air on the strongest possible forced expiration through a wide nozzle. See also chapter 6.

Percussion A method used in examining the chest or the abdomen. A finger of one hand is pressed firmly on the part of the body being examined and tapped briskly with the tip of a finger of the other hand. The quality or resonance of the sound produced indicates whether the underlying area is air-filled, fluid-filled or solid. In many people with asthma the chest is found to be abnormally resonant (hyper-resonant) on percussion. This is because, as a result of the increased difficulty in breathing out, more air than normal is retained in the lungs.

Phagocyte An amoeba-like cell of the **immune system** that responds to contact with a foreign object, such as a bacterium, by surrounding, engulfing and digesting it. Phagocytes occur widely throughout the body wherever they are likely to be required. Some wander freely throughout the tissues.

Prostaglandins A group of fatty acid hormones that occur throughout the tissues and body fluids. They are produced from cell membrane fats by the action of an enzyme. They have many different actions. Some of them cause asthma symptoms; some relieve them. Some cause narrowing of arteries; some widen them. Some promote blood clotting; some reduce it. They commonly stimulate pain nerve endings; some induce abortion; some reduce stomach acid secretion. Painkilling drugs such as aspirin act by preventing the release of prostaglandins from injured tissue.

Proteins Large molecules made up of tens to thousands of amino acids linked together. These long chains of amino acids are often folded in specific ways. The body is largely made up of fibrous, insoluble proteins, such as collagen. Globular proteins are soluble and include the enzymes, many of the hormones and the blood proteins such as haemoglobin and the immunoglobulins (antibodies).

Radioactive tracer A biochemcial substance in which atoms of one kind are mildly radioactive so that their movement and destinations can be detected. The use of these tracers is invaluable in medical research.

Reactivity A term much used in the asthma literature to refer to the tendency of the muscles in the walls of the air tubes to contract under the influence of various triggers – such as pollen grains or house dust mite excreta – that have no effect on non-asthmatic people.

Rebound phenomenon The proneness of certain drugs, especially air tube wideners (bronchodilators), to work well for a time and then to produce an increased tendency to cause the opposite effect (increased **reactivity**).

Rhonchi Continuous wheezing sounds of low or high pitch heard with a stethoscope when listening to the breathing sounds. Rhonchi are caused by partial obstruction of the smaller breathing tubes in the lungs (bronchioles) by narrowing, swelling of the lining or partial obstruction by thick mucus. Rhonchi are characteristic signs of an asthmatic attack.

Rotacaps Capsules of medication used with the **Rotahaler**.

Rotahaler An inhaler device for dry powder, dispensed in two-colour capsules. One of these is inserted, as instructed, into the end of the device. The 'rota-' refers to the fact that rotation of the outer sleeve of the inhaler breaks off the inner half of the powder capsule, releasing the powder into the interior of the device. The current of air produced by the inhalation through the device then carries the powder into the air passages. Rotahaler devices, and the associated rotacap capsules, must be kept completely dry. If damp, the powder clumps into particles too large to be inhaled.

Salbutamol One of the principal drugs used in the treatment of asthma. Salbutamol relaxes the **smooth muscle** in the walls of the air tubes – i.e. it is a bronchodilator drug. It is also used to treat chronic bronchitis and emphysema. It can be taken by inhalation or by mouth or, in severe cases, by slow injection directly into a vein.

Smooth muscle The kind of involuntary muscle occurring in the walls of the air tubes of the lungs, in the walls of blood vessels, the intestines and in the bladder. Smooth muscle is controlled by the **autonomic nervous system** and by various hormones and drugs acting through receptor sites on the muscle cell walls. It is called 'smooth' because, unlike the muscle under voluntary control, it is seen to be unstriped when examined under a microscope.

Sodium cromoglycate One of the principal drugs used in the treatment of asthma. The mode of action of cromoglycate is not well understood, but its effect is to reduce the tendency for **mast cells** to **degranulate**. See also chapter 7.

Spinhaler A dry powder inhaler of a slightly more complex design than the **Rotahaler**. See chapter 8 for details.

Sulphur dioxide One of the common atmospheric pollutants that results mainly from industrial activities, especially power generation. Sulphur dioxide is highly toxic and interferes with the action of **cilia**. As a result, allergens such as pollen grains and fungal spores remain longer in contact with the lung tissues. The increasing atmospheric levels of sulphur dioxide are thought to be one of the causes of the steady rise in the prevalence of asthma.

T lymphocytes See **T cells.**

T cells One of the two great divisions of lymphocytes which are the central operators of the immune system of the body. Some T cells are killer (cytotoxic) cells and attack foreign material such as viruses directly. Others are **helper cells**.

Theophylline An air tube-widening (bronchodilator) drug used to treat asthma. Trade names are Choledyl, Labophylline, Lasma, Nuelin SA, Slo-Phyllin, Theo-Dur, Uniphyllin Continus and Franol. The latter also contains **ephedrine**. Theophylline can be taken by mouth or can be given by slow injection into a vein.

Trachea The windpipe. The trachea divides into the right and left main bronchus and these in turn divide into numerous smaller branches.

Trigger Any substance or agency that can start up an asthmatic attack.

Urticaria Nettle rash or hives. An allergic skin condition featuring itchy, raised, pink areas surrounded by pale skin. These patches persist for periods of half an hour to several days and then disappear. Urticaria may result from sunlight, cold, food, or drug allergy, insect bites, scabies, jelly fish stings or contact with plants. Treatment is with antihistamine drugs or corticosteroids. Urticaria is one of the features of **atopy**.

Vital capacity The volume of air that can be expelled from the lungs by a full effort following a maximal deep breath.

Xanthine drugs The important class of drugs used to treat asthma that include aminophylline and theophylline. Caffeine and theobromine are also xanthines but are of no value in the treatment of asthma.

References

Allergy immunology and asthma, *JAMA*, 25 November 1992.
Asthma: and cross-country skiers, *BMJ* (20 November 1993), p. 1326.
and heparin, *NEJM* (8 July 1993), pp. 90, 129.
and the atmosphere, *BMJ* (10 September 1994), p. 619.
and the bean, *Lancet* (3 September 1989), p. 538.
assessment, *JRSM* (June 1994), p. 330.
control with aerosols, *NEJM* (2 October 1986), pp. 870, 888.
difficult cases, *BMJ* (16 September 1989), p. 695.
drugs – the risks, *New Sci* (6 April 1991), p. 17.
education, *BMJ* (26 February 1994), p. 568.
has prevalence increased? *BMJ* (19 May 1990), p. 1306.
hospital admission, *BMJ* (28 March 1992), p. 819.
in childhood, *BJHM* (20 January 1993), p. 127.
in childhood, epidemiology, *BMJ* (18 June 1994), p. 1548.
in childhood: prevalence, severity, *JAMA* (18 November 1992), p. 2673.
in children: current concepts, *NEJM* (4 June 1992), p. 1540.
in school children, *Pract* (8 September 1989), p. 1174.
injected steroids, *Lancet* (24 August 1991), p. 479.
major scientific coverage, *New Sci* (13 February 1993), p. 38.
management, *BJHM* (2 February 1994), p. 80; *RIP* (December/January 1990), pp. 20, 26.
management of acute attack, *Lancet* (18 January 1986), p. 131.
medical progress, *NEJM* (31 December 1992), p. 1928.
peak flow meters, *BMJ* (26 February 1994), pp. 548, 564.
salmeterol, salbuterol, *NEJM* (12 November 1992), p. 1420.
self-management, *BMJ* (26 February 1994), pp. 547, 556, 559.
tolerance to beta agonists, *Lancet* (2 October 1993), pp. 818, 833.
treatment, *BMJ* (29 June 1991), p. 1599.
treatment in small children, *BMJ* (16 July, 1988), p. 154.
treatment symposium, *BJCP Supplement*, 67, March 1989.
treatment update, *BJPP* (November 1990), p. 372.
why do people get it? *BMJ* (2 October 1993), p. 813.
Asthma allergy and sex, *BJSM* (February 1989), p. 69.

Beta-2 agonists in asthma, *BMJ* (24 September 1994), p. 794.
Betel-nut chewing and asthma, *Lancet* (9 May 1992), p. 1134.
Budesonide in asthma, *NEJM* (15 September 1994), pp. 700, 737.
Car emission triggers asthma attacks, *New Sci* (1 October 1994), p. 4.
Causation of asthma, *Lancet* (29 May 1993), p. 1369.
Cyclosporin treatment of asthma, *Lancet* (8 February 1992), pp. 324, 338.
Death from asthma, *NEJM* (12 May 1994), p. 1383.
Oral steroids for asthma, *JAMA* (14 October 1992), p. 1926.
Drug treatment of asthma: new approach, *NEJM* (30 November 1989), p. 1517.
Exercise and asthma, *NEJM* (20 August 1987), p. 502.
Exercise-induced asthma, *NEJM* (12 May 1994) p. 1362.
Gene for IgE receptor and asthma, *New Sci* (11 June 1994), p. 183.
Growing up with asthma, *BMJ* (9 July 1994), pp. 72, 90.
Heroin and asthma, *BMJ* (10 December 1988), p. 1511.
Large-volume spacers in asthma, *BMJ* (12 September 1992), p. 598.
Magnesium and asthma, *Lancet* (6 August 1994), p. 357.
Mechanism of allergic asthma, *Lancet* (7 March 1992), pp. 569, 584.
Mite antigen and asthma, *Lancet* (13 October 1990), p. 895.
Nose and asthma, *Lancet* (23 April 1994), p. 991.
Ozone and asthma, *Lancet* (27 July 1991) pp. 199, 211.
Respiratory viruses and asthma, *BMJ* (16 October 1993), p. 982.
Risk of fatal asthma, *JAMA* (23 December 1992), p. 3462.
Salbutamol in asthma, *Lancet* (4 June 1994), p. 1379.
Salmeterol versus steroids in asthma, *Lancet* (23 July 1994), p. 219.
Salmeterol versus salbuterol in asthma, *BMJ* (17 April 1993), p. 1034.
Salt and asthma, *BMJ* (6 November 1993), p. 1159.
Steroid tapering in asthma, *Lancet* (6 February 1993), p. 324.
Steroids in asthma, *Lancet* (5 December 1992), p. 1384.
Treating childhood asthma in Singapore, *BMJ* (14 May 1994), p. 1282.
Treating mild asthma, *NEJM* (15 September 1994), p. 737.
Unstable asthma and theophylline, *BMJ* (23 November 1991), p. 1317.
Ventilatory support in asthma, *BJHM* (3 March 1993), p. 357.
Yoga and asthma, *Lancet* (9 June 1990), p. 1381.

Key to journals

JAMA	Journal of the American Medical Association
BMJ	British Medical Journal
NEJM	New England Journal of Medicine
Lancet	The Lancet
JRSM	Journal of the Royal Society of Medicine
New Sci	New Scientist
BJHM	British Journal of Hospital Medicine
Pract	The Practitioner
RIP	Respiratory Diseases in Practice
BJCP	British Journal of Clinical Practice
BJPP	British Journal of Pharmaceutical Practice
BJSM	British Journal of Sexual Medicine

Useful addresses

The National Asthma Campaign
Providence House
Providence Place
London N1 0NT
Helpline (local call rate) Telephone: Linkline 0345 010203
General enquiries Telephone: 0171 226 2260

British Thoracic Society
78 Hatton Garden
London EC1
Telephone: 0171 831 8778

British Wellness Council
70 Chancellors Road
London W6 9RS
Telephone: 0181 741 1231

Health and Safety Executive
Rose Court
2 Southwark Bridge
London SE1 9HS
Telephone: 0171 717 6000

Department of Health
Health Information Services
Telephone: Freephone 0800 66 55 44

The Asthma and Allergy Foundation of America
1125 15th Street NW, Suite 502
Washington DC 20005

The American Lung Association
1740 Broadway
New York, NY 10019

Index